Prostate Cancer Adventures

A Forthright and Humorous Tale of My Prostate Cancer Treatments

Published by Amazon.

Prostate Cancer Adventures: A Forthright and Humorous Tale of My Prostate Cancer Treatments

ISBN. 9781708713690

Prostate Cancer Adventures is available for sale at:
    www.amazon.com

Cover Design and Layout by Michael Sisti

Readers' Comments

"Overall, this book is a cross between the best of Dave Barry and Tales from the Crypt."

"Your unflinching detail and honest rendition of your experience is remarkable."

"My father contracted prostate cancer which ultimately led to his demise, partly due to the less refined diagnostic and treatment options back then but also he lacked the kind of candid information you provide in your book. He was a reticent person and discussing health concerns much less anything below the belt was difficult for him -- like your ancestry. I think had he been able to read what you have written he would have benefited greatly."

"Reading the section on "Getting the fluid drinking right" had me running to the bathroom in some kind of urinary empathy."

"The book includes lots of medical things I never knew (e.g., Gleason score, regeneration of healthy cells following radiation) but for me the gold in the book is the nitty gritty of the experience."

"I have a lovely image of you hunched over the commode trying for that bowl movement, farting on command for the MRI test (I'm practicing that) and learning to cope with hot flashes. One thing perhaps is to know about these things, but quite another is to have them brought to life with such immediacy."

"I thought the book would be a great help to anyone going through both the prostate surgery and recurrence - especially the practical advice and what you thought when you heard the news at various steps in the process."

"Men need pals and good laughs to get through really scary medical challenges like prostate cancer. The author gives us the inside story with humor, honesty, and perspective so we can face such challenges with fortitude and optimism. A must read for male patients and their friends, family, and care providers."

"I have taken the liberty of forwarding this book to both George Lucas and Steven Spielberg. You may be asked to rewrite it as a script. I suggested George Clooney play you and Nicole Kidman your wife. On a serious note I hope you can get this into wider circulation as I think it would be extraordinarily helpful to many, many men and their families."

Dedication

This book is dedicated to millions of men who have, are currently experiencing or will experience prostate cancer in the future. The book is intended to inform men of the various issues they will face as they endure either surgical removal of the prostate or radiation therapy to kill the cancer. I first had the surgery and then, with a recurrence, also had the standard radiation treatment, together with hormone treatment. Most of the issues the book discusses are not addressed in the various web sites on prostate cancer nor are they fully explained by doctors and nurses.

Book Overview

As men age, the topic of prostate issues becomes a part of nearly every conversation. Unfortunately, the comments shared are usually based on hearsay, rather than fact. And this leads to confusion, rather than knowledge. In this book, Allan Odden provides a clear description of his own experiences dealing with this potentially life-threatening affliction. And he does it in a substantive way using an entertaining and humorous style, making this authoritative book a must read for all men over forty.

Table of Contents

Foreword

On December 31, 2018, I received positive confirmation that my prostate cancer had returned, called a recurrence in the field. In early June of that year, I had a prostatectomy, i.e., surgery to remove my prostate. This capped five years of a rising PSA count, an MRI that showed cancer was likely in the prostate, a biopsy that confirmed that was the case, and surgical removal of the organ.

After successful surgery (or radiation), the PSA count is supposed to drop to zero, or to <0.05. Mine didn't. A month after surgery, my PSA dropped, but only to 0.12. Two months later it dropped further to 0.10, a good sign. But then a month later, when I had my four-month after surgery visit with my urologist and surgeon, the PSA had risen to 0.11. He said, "Let's give it another couple of months and hope it resumes a downward trek."

So, 1 left Chicago for Sarasota, where my wife and I spent the winter. In early December, I went to one of the Quest Diagnostics Labs in Sarasota and ordered the PSA test; the result was a PSA of 0.21. The urology nurse in Chicago said the high number could be caused by a difference in how that lab worked from the one at Northwestern Memorial Hospital where I was getting my treatments. I said I'd be in Chicago for New Year's Eve and she said to get a PSA test in the Northwest lab when I arrived. I did.

At 4 pm on New Year's Eve, the nurse called with the results: a PSA count of 0.21. She said, "You need to see the radiation oncologist."

What a message to receive on the cusp of New Year's Eve. I was shaking. Everything had gone well with the surgery, and I was fully recovered. But the cancer was still inside me. Why had I gone through all the agony of the surgery just to be back where I started? Would I make it through this second treatment? Would I die before I thought I would? And I dreaded radiation, which I knew was a Monday through Friday event for eight weeks, with possible unpleasant side effects. I was bummed.

This book is a forthright, factual and detailed account of what I experienced over a 12-month period. I had wonderful medical treatment from the Northwestern Medical Group and super emotional support from family and many friends across the country, including several who also have struggled with prostate cancer. My wife, Eleanor, was a rock and supported me at every turn in the road, several of which impacted her as well.

At every step of the way, however, I encountered things that I did not know, procedures the medical community did not explain fully at least to my understanding, and situations that were only vaguely informed by reading the Internet. Each step of the journey tested the power of my self-confidence and strength of my emotional being. My hope is that by laying out what I experienced in detailed and – at times – humorous ways, those going through the prostate cancer experience in the future will be better prepared than I was.

I can also say that as I told friends and family that I had prostate cancer, I learned that many of them had also had the same malady. I guess we men don't talk about these things as much as we should, especially when they concern our groin area. But the most comforting words for me during my journey came from friends and family who shared their experiences in detail with me. I cannot emphasize enough how much those shared experiences meant to me; I knew I was not alone, and I felt their compassion and understanding.

So, for those of you who must go through the prostate cancer journey, I hope reading this book will help you on your journey. And I also urge you to reach out and find people whom you can talk to. You will become part of a supportive community, and you will thank God for that community's gift of emotional strength and courage to face your challenge head on with dignity, and to be better prepared at each step for what might happen.

You must understand this journey concerns basically elements that are part of a man's genitals and sex life, with every issue laid bare, if you will. Procedures are provided by young, mainly female, and usually quite attractive nurses and technicians, with whom you also have multiple conversations you might not have very often, if ever, even with your wife. So, while my journey provided multiple opportunities to shed any thread of privacy or modesty, it also provided opportunities for humorous commentary. As you read about all my treatments, envision very good-looking young females providing them. At the same time, their age and attractiveness had no relationship to how the treatments were provided, which was efficient, effective, empathetic and to the highest levels of professionalism. In addition, at various points I have taken some literary prerogative to slightly exaggerate a point or inject a risqué inference, either to make it humorous or to emphasize it more. But mostly this is a factual portrayal.

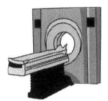

1

Introduction

When I wrote this account, I was a 75, almost 76-year-old Caucasian male. Furthermore, I thought I was three-fourths Norwegian, and one-eighth German and Russian.

Family Ethnic Background

My mother's parents were both full-blooded Norwegians. At the turn of the 19th century at the age of 19, they both left a Norway in depression and ended up in Duluth, Minnesota, my maternal grandmother via Canada and my maternal grandfather via New York.

My father's father, my paternal grandfather, was also Norwegian. My paternal grandfather was born in the United States after his mother and father had emigrated to the U.S. from Norway in the late 19th century. I think some of my simple, straight forwardness derives from this side of the family as my grandfather had a brother whose name was Knute Knute Odden (easier to remember two rather than three different names) and their father also was Knute Knute Odden, respectively called K.K. Odden. The son was K.K. Junior. This side of the family followed the KISS principle: Keep It Simple, Stupid.

I could have been KK the fourth. Thank God my grandparents and parents stopped that practice and gave me a real name. Although, I was called Oddball in college. Just after college in the mid-60s, I married my wife whose last name was Rubottom. That was a time when the feminist movement was in full-bore and women were reluctant to take on the man's last name after marriage; we toyed with merging our names, but then we'd be called the OddBottoms, so we dropped that idea pretty quickly. But I digress.

The lineage of my father's mother is a bit more complicated. She was Jewish and had both a Russian and German background. Her mother's family left Eastern Russia during the pogroms directed toward Jews in the latter part of the 19th century. Her father left Germany about the same time. Both parents ended up in New York where my paternal grandparents were born. He was a tailor. Max and Minnie Mogilner were married, started a family, and then for God knows what reason, moved to Duluth, Minnesota, where the average balmy day was, and still is, only 50 degrees.

Actually at that time, Duluth was one of the most prosperous cities in the country, located at the foot of the Mesabi and Virginia iron ranges, with train after train bringing all that rich iron ore to the Duluth harbor, where it was loaded onto the long, sleek iron ore boats, which braved the Great lakes of Superior, Michigan and Huron to deliver that "rust-colored gold" to the industrial Midwest cities of Chicago, Gary (IN), and Pittsburgh. Lore had it that in the 1920s and 1930s the city of Duluth had one of the highest concentrations of millionaires in the country.

I'd always wanted to know, though, if that 3/4, 1/8 and 1/8 breakdown of my ethnic background was actually true. So I was delighted when, during one of my first appointments with my urologist (to whom I had been referred after a rising PSA count), a graduate student approached me and asked if I'd be willing to be part of study that was being conducted seeking to find factors that caused or were correlated with prostate cancer. Being a former professor and knowing the hoops (human subjects' approval) the graduate student and her professor had to have jumped through to get this study approved, I immediately said yes.

So, she took down my background information and then took a blood sample. Not being full-fledged nurse, she had to poke around quite a bit because it is difficult to get a needle into any of my veins. That has always been the case. By the time she had successfully inserted the needle, she was starting to sweat, blood was running around the crook in my arm, and I was wondering why I had agreed to be a study subject. The sight of blood now makes me feel faint, and here I was, nervous as hell about the possible prostate cancer, and getting my arm all bloody for a bloody study by some professor!

The upside, I guess the incentive for my doing this, was that I would learn more about my genealogical background, something about which as I said was intriguing to me. The graduate student gave me her card and said I'd hear the results in 3-4 months. After 6 months, I gave her a call. Of course, no one answered so I left a message something like, "This is Allan Odden. Are the genealogical results forthcoming sometime soon?"

I didn't get a call back very quickly.

About a month later, I did get a call. But then I was busy, probably playing golf. After the round was over, I called her back and she said,

"The results will be here in about another month or two."

I was beginning to wonder now. If you take a swab of the inside of your mouth, and send it off to 23andMe, you get the results in 4-5 weeks. It was now well over 6 months and I was questioning whether the data would ever appear. On the other hand, maybe the study was getting very detailed ethnic information, and it was taking a long time to conduct those more specific analyses.

Finally, about two months later I received an envelope from Northwestern Memorial Hospital (I was in the Northwestern University Memorial Medical Group). I quickly ripped open the envelope and took out the paper inside. It had the results: 97 percent European, 2 percent Native American (where did that come from?) and 0.01 percent Negroid – the latter of which is something most people get showing that we all derive from that one woman in central Africa. And I thought the latter figure was pretty cool: I came from the same place as everyone else in the world. I had no clue about the roots of the Native American percentage, which remain a mystery to me.

What a disappointment for the European results. I already knew I was "European." I wanted a break down like my adopted son had received. He was born to Korean parents on Cheju Island, which is off the southeast corner of South Korea. Several years ago, he had ordered a 23andMe analysis and received a disaggregated percentage breakdown of Asian: Korean (the highest percentage which made him happy), Japanese, Chinese and other South East Asian.

I was hoping for something along the same lines, perhaps percentages Scandinavian, German, Russian, maybe even further disaggregated to Norwegian,

Swedish, Finnish and Danish. Perhaps even some English and French if any of my Scandinavian ancestors had played around a bit or brought back to Norway a captive female after one of the Viking ravages in northern Europe. But no such luck in terms of the ethnic breakdown. In terms of playing around, the picture below of my great grandparents from Norway shows that my closest ancestors found it difficult to smile let alone play around! I was just predominately or virtually all European, which also includes western

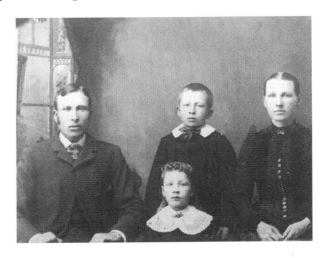

Russia by the way, even though most Russians want to be just Russian, and neither European nor Asian.

On the other hand, maybe some Vikings (Leif Ericson?) from long ago sailed to America, had relations with some Native Americans, and brought those offspring home, one of whom became part of my family tree! That would be pretty awesome, right? At least that is a possible explanation for the 2 percent Native American.

At any rate, there could be a connection between my prostate cancer and my ethnic background, as one element of the study was assessing whether ethnic background had any correlation to the emergence of prostate cancer. But I certainly hoped that the study was getting categories more precise than those sent to me. What good would a correlation between prostate cancer and continents (Europe in my case) be?

But let's go back to the beginning and let me tell you how my prostate journey began to unfold.

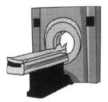

2

The Onset

I had always been healthy, luckily. But my family health background was a bit iffy.

Family Health Background

My father died of a heart attack at 55, his brother died of a heart attack at 65, and their father – my grandfather –also died of a heart attack at 65. So, I had heart attacks on my father's side of the family.

My mother lived to age 95. But her dad died of cancer at age 70 and her mother died of cancer at the age of 59. So, I had cancer on my mother's side.

Not exactly an enviable family medical background. I always wondered how long I would live. Would I make it past my 50s? Would I make it past my 60s? Not many in the family had, although by the time I was in my 50s, my mother was doing well in her 70s, as were her two brothers, one of whom including my mother lived well into his 90s. But I didn't know that then.

So, when I entered my 50s, and my kids were then only 13 and 9, I began to worry; I never really told anyone, but I started wondering if my time would soon be up. When I'd see my doctor, he'd always say my health indicators looked really good and all the numbers were in the normal range. I'd respond with a muted comment. One day when I was in my mid-50s, he looked at me and said,

"Allan, you are in excellent health. All your numbers are good; though your cholesterol is high normal, it is stable and has been at that level for years. There is nothing wrong with you – well, you could lose ten pounds but .... There is every indication that you will live for many more years. Cheer up. Many patients your age have many issues. You don't. You aren't taking any drugs, not even a statin. You should have many good years in front of you."

Those comments made a difference and I took them to heart. From that day on I began to act as if I'd live to a ripe old age. And when I hit 60 and took the medical exam for a ten-year- life insurance policy spanning my age from 60 to 70, a nurse came and did all the tests, said everything looked really good, even my low blood pressure. Then she asked what medicines I was taking. I said none, other than a Benadryl at night to help with sleep.

She looked up and said, "No meds?"

And I said, "No, none."

"Viagra?" she asked.

And I said, "No, not yet anyway."   She responded, "First time in my life for a 60-year-old."

And that made me feel even more confident and actually a bit cool – I did have excellent health and so far, didn't need Viagra.

My health stayed that way throughout my 60s.

Just before I hit 70, I decided to retire from my job at the University of Wisconsin-Madison. I had worked 50 years, 20 years there, 9 years at the University of Southern California, and 21 years at other places including public school teaching in New York City. I had published 275 articles and written 35 books and manuscripts, had raised an average of a million research dollars a year for research over my 29 years of university work, and felt it was time to shed the day job. I would continue consulting for state legislatures as they sought to make public school funding more adequate and more equitable, but that work was intermittent and it was time to enjoy my last years, however long they would last.

Rising PSA

That year, 2013, when I had my annual physical my doctors asked me if I wanted a PSA test. I had it in 2011 and it was 1.4, well within the normal range of 0-4 for a man of my age.

I said, "Why ask me?"

He said, "Well, if it is rising, I'm not sure what I'd tell you as there is no really good result from treatment; everyone pretty much gets some level of incontinence and impotence if they need treatment for prostate cancer. And the medical recommendation these days is that men 70 or older do not need to get their PSA; if they have prostate cancer, which most men do by the time they die, it is usually very slow growing, so most men outlive it. And there are too many false positives from the PSA test. Too many men see a rising PSA, get the prostate surgically removed or radiated, and have some degree of incontinence and impotence when they really didn't have a cancer that would grow and thus needed to be treated."

That was a bit of disturbing news, and I didn't relish having either incontinence or impotence, but being a data guy, I nevertheless said, "Yah, I want the PSA test."

And I got it. And the PSA was higher than it ever had been. It was only 2.53 but it was now on a rising trend.

So, the first days of my retirement, I get indicators that I could be getting prostate cancer. I was both pissed and nervous. Knowing I will die sometime, I didn't want it to happen to me now, just shortly after I had fully embraced my up-to-then good health and decided I was going to live for many more years. And I had worked a long time and wanted to enjoy some retirement years, even if at some point I'd need medication to get solidly excited (get my play on words?)! But the results were a kick in the gut. Something was going on. And it wasn't good.

Moving on Our Retirement

Nevertheless, my wife and I moved forward with our retirement plans. We sold our downtown condominium in Madison (WI), we sold our modest vacation place in Wildwood (FL), which by then had become the southern border of the huge Villages Development in central Florida. (Today, The Villages is a 55+ community of over 100,000 people, all of whom are enjoying and active retirement, as well as an active sex life as it has one of the highest concentrations of sexually transmitted diseases (STDs) of any community in the country. It's about bout 90 percent Republican and super conservative, but I guess they like to play around, as it were.)

We decided to have our northern base in Chicago, where in 2000 we had purchased an apartment in the historic Edgewater Beach Apartments (EBA), a 20 story apartment building designed by Benjamin Marshall, who in the 1920s also had designed the Edgewater Beach Hotel (now demolished), the first modern downtown hotel – the Drake, and several other iconic, downtown Chicago buildings. The building was on Sheridan Road with just a public park between it and picturesque Lake Michigan. Though the dream of most people in Wisconsin was to acquire a cabin on some lake farther north in the state and get away from all the "urban noise" of Madison, we were city people. We had lived in New York, Denver, and Los Angeles, had close relatives in Dallas and Houston, and while Madison was a grand mid-sized city, we and our kids loved big cities. Further, our son, Robert, had also now made Chicago his home.

We bought a 2-bedroom unit in EBA in 2000. When we told friends in Madison, most looked at us like we had lost our mind. It was the exact opposite of what they wanted. By about the fifth such reaction, we simply said, "Well, that is our cabin on the lake," as we had a beautiful view of Lake Michigan from several windows in our apartment. And folks nodded; at least they knew we had a decent reason for wanting to be in the city. In 2006, we moved inside the building to a somewhat larger unit on a higher floor, and even had our son living in a separate unit in the same building for several years. It had become our northern home.

We also moved our Florida base to Sarasota, which is the cultural center of the southwestern Florida coast. It has a symphony, an opera, a ballet, many theaters, scores of restaurants, the number one beach in America – Siesta Key Beach – and golf courses galore. We found a home on the eighth fairway in a place called Misty Creek, which was developed in the 1990s and 2000s in a nature preserve on the outskirts of the city. Indeed, half the holes of the golf course are in the preserve, and there is wildlife galore – sand hill cranes, great blue herons, egrets, ibis, anhingas, cormorants, osprey, eagles, deer, as well as alligators – all around and on the golf course, and the homes as well. We loved it.

The day we moved in we said to each other, "Hey, if we get ten good years here that will be terrific. We'd then both be 80, and life would have treated us pretty well."

The next summer, when I had my physical, my PSA had risen to above 3.

Beginning Retirement

We initially thought we would find our health care providers in Sarasota, as we could no longer use the HMO we had used during the 20 years we lived in Madison. But getting new doctors in Sarasota is not easy; hundreds of families move there every year and there is usually a six month or so time period before a doctor will see a new patient. Most of the newcomers are seniors on Medicare so do not add much to a doctor's bottom line, until they need lots of care.

I asked fellow golfers in our new community to recommend a doctor, identified a group that sounded like they did a good job and were affiliated with the highly rated Sarasota Memorial Hospital, and made an appointment to see an internist in January of 2015.

Unfortunately, my 95-year-old mother became quite ill in early January of 2015 and died in the middle of the month. For the past three years I had talked with her on the telephone nearly every day, usually when I was taking my morning 4-mile walk. But she had been too sick the last couple of weeks and we had not talked. When my sister told me she and my other siblings had called in hospice, I immediately flew to Minneapolis to be with my mother for her last days.

While there, I called the doctor's office in Sarasota, told them I could not make the appointment as I was in Minnesota where my mother was dying, and asked if I could push the appointment to the end of the month. They said, "No. You'll have to wait another six months." That sort of pissed me off. I guess they didn't care what caused my delay. An appointment for a new patient was simply six months out, regardless of the context.

So, I decided to try and get an appointment with the internist my wife had seen in the Northwestern Medical Group affiliated with Northwestern Memorial Hospital in Chicago. I was going to spend a couple of weeks in Chicago after my mother's service, to spend some time with my son who was still living there and to watch the Super Bowl with him, which was won by the Seattle Seahawks, quarterbacked by Russell Wilson who had spent a spectacular nine months at Madison a couple of years previously. The doctor's office said, no problem, we can get you in the last week of January.

So, after my mother's service, I traveled to Chicago, watched the Super Bowl with my son, celebrated the Seahawks' Super Bowl win, met my new doctor, had my annual physical – now called the annual wellness visit – including the full blood test, as well as the PSA test.

The result: PSA was 4.29.

What is a Normal PSA?

The doctor said that was still close to the normal range for a man of my age – now to be 72 in the fall – and that we should continue to watch the number until it got higher.

I said fine.

But I've always wondered what the "normal range" PSA means for men, especially men over 70. Does that include all men, men without prostate cancer, whose PSA would be close to zero (unless he had free prostate specific antigens, more on this later), as well as men with prostate cancer whose PSA could be any number? I didn't and still do not know a good answer to that question. Personally, I'd like a better description of the normal range, and what "normal" means. Save for the existence of "free antigens," which can only be identified in a more complex PSA analysis that is not normally conducted, a prostate cancer free man should have a PSA count of 0 or close to 0. Something higher means there is something going on which is increasing the PSA count, perhaps a rise of the "free antigens," maybe an enlarged prostate (which can be felt with the digital test – you know when the doc sticks his finger up your rectum and feels around, sometimes using an additional finger to get a second opinion), trauma, infection or – the onset of prostate cancer.

From what I have read on the Web, the normal high-level PSA for men below 60 years of age is 4; any PSA above that would be referred to as an "elevated PSA." From 60 to 70, the high normal figure rises to 4.5. And by age 70 it is about 6.5. Though I'd be concerned if it was 6.5, even if the docs would say that is high normal.

But a PSA at my level – then 4.29 – was referred to as an "elevated PSA," and, as far as I was concerned, that was not good, even though I did not know whether it was "bad." Indeed, I had recently been turned down for long term care insurance because of an "elevated" PSA level.

The point is that the PSA is only one indicator. There are cases of men having a PSA just above one who had prostate cancer with a Gleason of 7. Another friend of mine with a PSA well within the "normal" range for his age, had a family history of prostate cancer, so the doctor ordered a biopsy and found cancer with a Gleason of 7.0. Each man and his doctor need to determine how to address possible prostate cancer when the PSA is something other than negligible. There are no pat answers.

Remember, this was still the period when the medical community was recommending that men over 70 did not need to worry about prostate cancer, as most would outlive the cancer even if it emerged in their body. So, I agreed to wait until the doctor thought the numbers suggested that I should see a urologist.

For some reason, I had another appointment in October of 2015 and the PSA had then risen to 5.04. The advice still was to not rush to judgment and to wait. The going theory for men of my age who had rising PSA scores, was that unless there was a dramatic change in the slope of the change, all should be OK. I did plot my PSA numbers and the slope was clearly rising, but I didn't know if the acceleration of the rise was "dramatic." So, I continued to wait.

Since that time I have read much more on the early signs of prostate cancer and have now concluded that if one's PSA rises to above 4 and there has been more than a 0.75 increase in the PSA over a two year time period, it would be wise to see a urologist. The rise could be caused by an enlarged prostate, by "free" antigens, by prostate cancer, and other issues, but in my view a prudent man would begin investigating these issues, and not wait for larger increases in the PSA.

Additional Health Issues

About that same time, I began to have what is called "discolored semen." How is that for a medical term? Given that my PSA was rising, and I knew that the prostate gland produced semen, I was a bit concerned. When I told my internist about the discolored semen, she was somewhat puzzled. So, who could tell me the meaning or importance of this phenomenon? Again, I looked it up on the web. Discolored semen can be caused by several factors, including cancer. Most articles referred to red or pink semen, which indicated blood was involved, a point my internist also made. Mine was neither but more a brownish color, not completely, but not the normal milky white. I never did get a good answer about that issue, but the web does indicate that discolored semen could be caused by prostate cancer, so there was another possible indicator of the onset of prostate cancer.

In addition, I also came face-to-face with another health reality of older men (as well as women). Every now and then my blood pressure, which always was quite low, tested higher than normal. And my cholesterol, though remaining at the high normal range, began to creep above that level. So, my doctor said that I should consider taking a statin. Being proud that I was taking virtually no meds, I reacted negatively, and said my health background is cholesterol at the high normal level, so there should be no worry.

In response, she politely stated, "Well, we have a risk factor formula; I just entered your data and you have a 25 percent chance of a cardiac event in the next ten years."

I looked at her thinking, "At 72 I probably have a 25 percent chance of dying in the next ten years."

But I kept those thoughts to myself. I did ask her what variables were in the formula. And she said, "Gender and age, which you cannot change. But it also includes blood pressure and the cholesterol reading, which you can change." And she argued that taking a statin usually had no downside effects and would simply improve my health condition. I acceded and began taking a statin and indeed my cholesterol is now much lower, around 160 with the good cholesterol high and the bad cholesterol low, so I am in a better condition. And I had no side effects from the statin.

There also is some evidence that statins lower the risk of prostate cancer, a point my internist did not make. But taking the statin could have helped reduced the severity of my prostate cancer.

A PSA Above 7

By the fall of 2017, though, when after my annual physical the PSA came back in excess of 7, above the high normal range for men of my age, my internist said it was now time for me to see the urologist. Gulp! Prostate cancer, incontinence, impotence – all could be in my future. UGH.

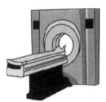

3

The Diagnosis

I immediately made an appointment to see the urologist, also in the Northwestern Medical Group associated with Northwestern Memorial Hospital.

Not Rushing into a Biopsy

His first comment was that we were not going to rush into conducting a biopsy. He said that while straightforward procedures, biopsies were body invasive and could cause harm, and there was no reason to do them just because of a rising PSA. Nowadays, he went on to say, there were several intervening steps taken before a biopsy was conducted, and those steps had dramatically reduced the false positives shown by just a rising PSA.

(The background here is that ten or so years ago, most doctors recommended a biopsy when the patient had a rising PSA. The biopsies included taking 12-14 random samples from the prostate, assuming that the large number of samples taken would show whether there was cancer in the prostate. Diagnostic tools today are much more advanced and precise, and, in my lay opinion, immediate biopsies and totally "random" biopsies should never be conducted.)

My urologist said the first step was to get a "free" PSA test. A "free" PSA test indicates whether the rise in the PSA count is due to "free antigens" (whatever they are) which are good, or cancer related antigens that attach themselves to proteins such as cancer, which are not good. Enlarged prostates often produce free antigens. The nurse drew a blood sample, and I was told to return in a week, which I did.

The result: I had virtually no free antigens and my PSA remained above 7 – far beyond the normal range. So, my antigens probably were of the "bad guy" type. ☹

Getting an MRI of the Prostate

The next step was an MRI. MRI, which stands for magnetic resonance imaging, is a radiology test that provides detailed, high quality pictures of the inside your body. Unlike X-rays or CT scans, an MRI scan does not use radiation to create images. It uses powerful magnets, radio waves, and a computer. For me, the MRI scan would provide detailed diagnostic, 3D images of my prostate – in approximately one-quarter inch thick slices. My MRI was conducted using a high-field scanner. These machines (similar to those pictured on the title page) have a small, narrow tube that moves over the table on which the patient lies, which can be uncomfortable for claustrophobic patients and cannot handle patients who weigh more than 300 lbs. When inside, I just closed my eyes and tried to sleep.

The doctor said that during the recent past the medical community had learned how to take clear and detailed MRIs of the prostate. The MRI would show whether there were possible cancer lesions in the prostate and, if so, it would then guide the biopsy, which would target the biopsy sampling to those lesion areas.

I had the MRI conducted the following week. Now, this was a straightforward procedure. I lay on a table around which a large metal machine rotated for about two hours – with 5 to 15-minute sessions for various pictures. The result would be a 3-D picture of my prostate.

On the evening for my MRI, I arrived unfortunately with gas in my lower intestines, which would obscure the MRI process. So, the technician said,

"You have some gas bubbles in your bowel; could you get rid of them?"

I'd been trying to pass that gas for the past two hours with no success and looked at her with a face like, "Right now, on demand? Are you kidding me?"

And she said, "Just try."

So, I pushed and pushed, trying not to poop at the same time, and low and behold, after a loud, gas-passing fart, she said, "We are now good to go."

After reviewing the results, the doctor reported that the MRI showed that there were two and possible three lesions in the prostate that could be cancerous so that he would proceed to the next step and do the biopsy. It was becoming pretty clear that I probably had prostate cancer. ☹

Getting the Biopsy

The biopsy was scheduled shortly thereafter. For me this procedure was virtually painless but can be embarrassing. You lie on your side, and the doctor and his two assistants (both male and female) insert some kind of probe into your rectum, and then, with the guidance of the MRI, take samples of your prostate where the possible cancer exists, meaning a needle of some sort gets quickly injected into and retrieved from the prostate to obtain the sample. For each sample, the doctor would say, "Ready," then I heard and felt the snap of the needle quickly first piercing the rectum, and then piercing and removing itself and the sample tissue from the prostate. The team sampled each of the three possible cancerous areas twice and then also took additional random samples in other areas of the prostate. I believe they took about 14 samples in all but 6 were targeted to the lesions identified by the MRI.

The Results of the Biopsy: Gleason of 7

A week later, near the middle of October 2017, my wife, Eleanor, accompanied me to the doctor's office to get the results. She brought a notebook and pen so she could take notes, as I was not in any condition to take notes and interested only in interacting with the doctor. We arrived for our appointment and were quickly led into one of the patient rooms. The doctor's nurse, who I have come to know and respect over the course of this journey and who is a skilled, knowledgeable and supportive person, first gave us an overview. Most of the samples proved negative. A few had a Gleason of 3 + 3 or a 6 but two had a Gleason of 3 + 4, or a 7. She went on to say that a 7 was sort of an in-between score, higher than a 6, which would lead to watchful waiting and no immediate treatment, and lower than an 8, which would require immediate action. Nevertheless, she said the Gleason was a level at which she and the doctor strongly recommended I get the prostate removed, saying,

"You want to get the cancer out. Late term prostate cancer is very painful, and you want to avoid that if at all possible."

When the doctor arrived, he provided the same analysis of the MRI results as the nurse and recommended treatment sooner rather than later – either surgical removal or radiation of the prostate.

Bummer. But first a technical comment on Gleason scores. The Gleason score indicates how fast a tumor is likely to grow or spread. Each sample is given a grade of 1-5, with 1 being an almost normal tissue sample and 5 being cancerous and aggressive. Because each sample might contain areas with different grades, the lab gives two grades for each sample, one for the most common grade in the sample and another for the second most common grade. The Gleason score is the combination of the two numbers. A Gleason of six (3 + 3) or less means there is cancer but it is less aggressive and will likely grow very slowly. The usual advice for a Gleason of 6 is to engage in "watchful waiting," that is to monitor – every six months or so – the cancer until the PSA reaches a much higher level and/or a higher Gleason score emerges. A Gleason of 7 means the cancer is likely to grow, slowly but still faster than a Gleason of 6. Parsing that number even more, moreover, a Gleason of 3 + 4 or 7 would indicate a cancer that would grow more slowly, i.e., is less aggressive, than a Gleason of 4 + 3. A Gleason of 8, 9 or 10 indicates a more aggressive cancer that should lead to immediate treatment.

As noted, my two Gleason scores were 3 + 4 or 7, just above a score that would merit watchful waiting. As stated, both the urologist and nurse recommended that I should not do watchful waiting and move on to a more aggressive strategy that involved removing the prostate through surgery or radiation. They suggested I consult with the radiation oncologist before choosing which option, but I had quickly decided on the surgery option (which you will learn was accidentally the wise choice for me).

Remember this was mid-October, about the time my wife and I usually left Chicago to spend the winter months in Sarasota. So, I asked if we needed to act right now or would it be unwise to wait a few months and do the operation at the beginning of the summer? The doctor assured me there would be very little material change in the next six months and to go ahead and enjoy the winter in Florida. Which we did.

A Bonus from the Urologist

At that same office visit, I broached the doctor about my erectile disfunction, specifically my difficulty in getting and maintaining a solid erection. I was now 20 years older than that previous time when I did not need any love-making assistance. When I said I was having difficulties "performing" in bed, the urologist said,

"No surprise for a man of your age, and I suggest you try Viagra."

He quickly wrote a prescription for ten pills a month, renewable each month for 11 months. I wasn't quite sure I needed ten pills a month – sex every three days? I hope you are not shocked to learn that sex every three days exceeded our actual practice. If I had sex that often at my age, I might have a heart attack, although sex frequency was not in that "risk analysis" my internist had earlier conducted for me! Maybe you have sex every three days, but not me – after all, I was 75 and not 25. But I didn't say anything and just thanked the doctor for the prescription.

After the meeting, Eleanor and I drove right to the neighborhood drug store and ordered the new blue pills. We had to wait for a while and when we returned, there was a long line of people picking up their meds, and more people just waiting for their meds in the pick-up area. We got to the head of the line and said,

"A prescription for Odden."

And the person behind the desk yelled back in a loud voice, "Oh, the Viagra."

We both wanted to hide someplace as half the crowd spun their head and stared at us. The pharmacist then said each pill was $60, so the tab would be $600! I was sort of stunned at the price – I'd be paying a large tab for sex in the future and would have to stop my every three day habit! I looked at my wife for direction about spending that large amount.

And she said, very affirmatively, "We need it."

Note the use of the pronoun "we!" This wasn't just about me; this was an expenditure for both of us. So, we paid the bill and hastened home.

We didn't try the pill right away because it was still soon after the biopsy and we had been told the prostate was pretty traumatized and any semen it produced would be quite bloody. Nevertheless, we both were a bit anxious to see if the pill – sildenafil by its generic name – would work. So, after a week we decided to give it a go. I popped the pill and went for my daily walk, as it takes about an hour for sildenafil to take effect. When I got home, Eleanor was in the bedroom and I walked in and let's just say I became proud as a peacock! The pill was having its effect and we engaged in the activity the pill was designed to enhance. And my body did produce a quite bloody semen sample, sort of a damper on the successful event.

You should know, though, that Viagra or sildenafil, had now become part of any medical background. So every time I have a doctor's appointment, when the nurse asks what medications I am taking, I say Benadryl, Vitamin D (my internist had also suggested I take that), and the statin – and then the nurse usually asks, again in a loud voice,

"Viagra, too, right?"

And I quietly say, "Yes."

One time I listed sildenafil, and she asked, again in a not so soft voice, "Isn't that Viagra?"

So at least in every medical office, that cat is out of the bag. Even when I went to my dermatologist in Florida for my annual skin cancer check, conducted by another super young and very attractive female, the first thing she checked with me was my list of meds, each of which she read off, including the sildenafil! So, there are no secrets in the doctor's office.

The fall of 2017 and winter of 2018 in Florida went well. During these months I did receive advice and counsel from friends.

Advice and Counsel from Friends

Prior to then, in 2011 – the year of my 50th high school reunion, I had connected with three of my high school buddies who also spent the winter in the southwest Florida area. Every month, I played golf with them. In January 2018, one of them, who had strong feelings about boosting one's auto-immune system to ward off illness and cancer, said very seriously,

"Well, you can kick cancer with AHCC or Noxy Lane 4, 3 grams a day," which includes a mushroom concoction that allegedly boosts the auto immune system. And he was very insistent.

I looked it up on the Web and most, if not all, articles were skeptical. One study did show a possible modest impact. A four-week regime was supposed to do the trick. I concluded there were no downsides to trying it, so I took the mushroom pills for 8 weeks, got a prescription to get another PSA, and the result came back above 7 – no impact. So, I didn't buy any more mushroom pills.

I also was able to talk with two other friends in Sarasota, one who had had his prostate removed a few years earlier and another who was scheduled for and did have the operation in January. I went to brunch with the first friend. He said not to wait and to have the operation as soon as possible. He said his went fine, and that he was now cancer free, i.e., his PSA was close to zero.

He did share an amusing story. In the process leading up to his surgery, he had one of the old-fashioned biopsies – the taking of 14 random samples. He had gone to visit his doctor who was part of the University of Vermont's health system. The doc asked if it was OK for resident doctors to watch the procedure. My friend said no problem. So, he undressed, put on the proverbial gown, and was ushered into the biopsy procedure room, which was surrounded by glass observation windows. In the windows were twenty of so medical residents, mostly women. After securing my friend to the table, the table rotated to upend my friend with his legs spread, thus allowing the doctor to obtain the biopsy samples. My friend hadn't realized he'd be this quickly exposed and to so many! My friend was glad he didn't bump into any of the residents after he left the building when the procedure was completed.

He also reminded me that without a prostate, the body produces no semen, which is the fluid in a man's ejaculation. He said sex was still good, but that I would have a "dry" ejaculation. I had read about that on the web as well. He did say you "came" but it was dry. At least I'd be alive and if all went well would still have a sex life!

The other friend also shared with me his experience leading up to scheduling the surgery in January. He came from a family with a prostate cancer history and was quite vigilant about watching his PSA. Even though his PSA was just over 4, given his medical background, his urologist said they should conduct a biopsy. They did and found several cancerous cells. And this friend did not want to wait and immediately scheduled the surgery.

His surgery was more difficult than mine. Before a prostatectomy, one is told to stop taking aspirin or any medication that is an anti-inflammatory in order to reduce blood loss during the procedure. My friend did just that. But then there was some confusion, so after the operation, when the standard practice is to administer an anti-inflammatory, to reduce inflammation and pain, he was not given any, as the resident thought he already was taking one. The result was he experienced significant pain for the first two days, which was unusual for a robotic prostatectomy. After discussing the ongoing pain with the doctor, the doctor looked at the chart and realized he was not getting the anti-inflammatory and ordered that it immediately be administered. As a result, the pain subsided, and he moved into a more normal – and pain free – recovery.

My wife and I had dinner with his wife and him four weeks after the surgery. He looked pretty gaunt and had lost several pounds. I thought to myself quietly that perhaps one upside benefit to the surgery that was in my future was that I could lose ten pounds, about which my doctors had been badgering me for years. Sad to say, that didn't happen.

Later, he and I were able to have many lunches when we shared the recovery process from the surgery, focusing on activities designed to regain control over the urethra sphincter, which is traumatized during prostate removal and unable to completely control urination afterwards, particularly for older men. More on this later, but this is a big deal! After getting the catheter removed after surgery regaining urination control IS the next big challenge.

I must say that these conversations with friends and family who had experienced prostate removal were very important to me. They provided information, support and inducted me into the – surprisingly large – community of men recovering from prostate surgery and cancer. And such support people and groups are worth their weight in gold. The operation, side effects and the fact of having cancer is problematic enough but to go through it alone makes it more difficult. Drawing support from these man-to-man conversations, which often were also opportunities for sharing wry humor about one's genital area, was crucial for me, and I'd guess important for any man going through this prostate cancer journey.

Having the surgery or prostatectomy was the next step. In April 2018, I called the nurse and scheduled the operation for June 5.

Surgery or Radiation

One final note. When the biopsy showed that I had cancers with a Gleason of 7 in my prostate and the doctor and nurse suggested I should treat the issue, they said I could opt for either surgery or radiation and urged me to talk with the radiation oncologist. But I had talked with several other men, all of whom had had successful surgery, and as stated earlier, had pretty much opted for surgery without thoroughly investigating the radiation option. I also was told by friends who either were about to have prostate surgery or had had it in the recent past, that not only was radiation an eight week event – you get a five minute zap Monday through Friday – for eight weeks, but if the radiation beam missed the prostate it usually hit the colon and I could end up needing a colostomy bag for the rest of my life. That was not a chance I wanted to take (though I have learned these problems occur much less frequently today as the radiation treatment has become more precise).

What I did not learn then, because I did not investigate the options thoroughly, were the next treatment options if there was a cancer recurrence – that is if the surgery or radiation was not completely effective and/or when the cancer returned for whatever reason. It turns out that for recurrence after surgery, both radiation and hormone therapy are options, which together have super high effectiveness ratings, but that for recurrence after radiation, only hormone therapy is possible, because one area of the body can be radiated only once. And hormone therapy, while highly effective, is not as effective as the combination of hormone and radiation therapy. (The relevance of this paragraph will become obvious in later chapters.) As it turned out, I luckily had chosen the surgery option.

However, the above are general comments. There are other treatments for prostate cancer outside of the standard prostatectomy and radiation. There also is a "salvage prostatectomy" after radiation but it is much harder to do and is not done very often. And there are other combinations of treatments. So once again, specific treatments must be discussed between the patient and his doctor(s).

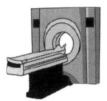

4

The Operation: Prostatectomy

We drove from Sarasota to Chicago in late May 2018, arriving just before Memorial Day. We had a week before I'd have my prostate removed. We celebrated our 52nd wedding anniversary on May 28.

We saw the doctor (my urologist who also would perform the surgery) several days before the procedure was scheduled. He and the nurse briefly described the robotic operation. YouTube has videos of these operations, both actual videos and animated videos. I watched the animated version, not having the stomach for the actual. The doctor said they would make six or so small slits across my lower stomach – groin area – two on the left, two in the middle and two on the right –

and then a larger slit just above the navel through which they would ultimately remove the prostate.

Prostatectomy

The operation consisted first of peeling the prostate away from the very sensitive nerves that surround the base of the penis where the prostate is located, very important nerves if you get my drift. Nerves that a man does not want damaged. Ok, fine. The doc said he'd be quite careful and had had very good success rates at preserving those nerves and assured me that nearly all his patients had "solid" use of those nerves after the surgery (after all, he thought I'd be using them 10 times a month!).

He said that next they would carefully cut around the prostate to detach it from all the surrounding tissue. But before they could remove the prostate, they would need to cut the urethra because it is embedded in the prostate. The urethra, i.e., the tube through which urine is eliminated from the body, runs from the bottom of the bladder, through the prostate, and on through the penis. I was starting to twitch a bit now, not knowing if this was "too much information" but understanding, a bit too clearly that there was going to be major "damage" not just to my groin region but to parts of my genitals, not the most pleasant thought.

To reattach the urethra, moreover, the doctor said they would "pull the bladder down" and reattach the two ends of the urethra where they had made the cut. Actually, he said it was a combination of pulling the bladder down and pulling the penis up in order to stitch the urethra back together. OMG, and he further said that there was a chance that I'd end up with a shorter penis – words that no sane man ever wants to hear! So, I was going to rid my body of prostate cancer, but there might be a price to pay. Ouch. Maybe I really wouldn't need those ten sildenafil pills every month after all! ☹

The weekend before the Tuesday surgery, my younger brother called, pretty teary eyed. He had just been diagnosed with stage 4 esophageal cancer, that had spread to his spine, liver and lungs. And his doctor had given him only a few months. He had always been an I-can-fix-anything kind of guy, but this news was beyond what he could fix. Even though he had golfed three weekends before, he was now in great pain and, as it turned out, had only a few weeks left. It was hard to talk, and though I wanted to immediately visit him, that was not possible as my surgery was imminent. This news made for a doubly troubled weekend before I had my cancer surgery so I would not have a similar stage 4 issue. It seemed our history of family cancer was catching up with us. ☹

Luckily, I was scheduled to be the first patient on Tuesday June 5. I arrived at the hospital at 6 A.M., got prepped and the team wheeled me into the operating room right about the scheduled time of 7 A.M. The doctor pointed out the Da Vinci Robot he would use for the operation. It was a rather large instrument, guided by joy sticks. Doing this operation was akin to playing a video game – with much higher stakes. Maybe all the video games young people play today are actually developing skills they will need in their professional work careers! I was transferred to the operating platform, the anesthesia was turned on, and I lost consciousness before I was able to reach 1 by counting backwards from 10.

I awoke in the recovery room about 11:30. I was ravenously hungry as I had stopped eating after lunch the day before. I asked if I could have something to eat and was given graham crackers. I immediately started eating them, but it was like devouring sand as my mouth was completely dry and I had no saliva. I was given water and after an hour or so my mouth had sufficient saliva for me to enjoy the crackers. Lunch also was served, and I ate every morsel.

Soon thereafter my wife, who had been informed at half hour intervals of my progress, was allowed to come and visit me. It was unusual for non-patients to be admitted to the recovery room, but a regular hospital room was not available at that time, and the medical team did not want her waiting any longer to see me. Her angelic smile was the tonic I needed at that time and I felt her warm embrace as she leaned over to kiss me. We didn't talk long but seeing her, if only briefly, was a high point for both her and me. She also was able to see me later in the afternoon when I was admitted to a room on a higher floor in the hospital.

Shortly before my wife was able to see me in the recovery room, the doctor and his team came to my bed. He said the operation went perfectly, no hitches. He felt my important nerves had been unharmed, which made me relax a bit. He further stated that there was no evidence of cancer in the lymph nodes, so the surgery team had left them alone. He did say that the cancer had grown some, causing a bulge in the prostate sac but that as far as they could tell, no cancer had escaped the prostate sac itself.

Then with a smile, he said, "You know that I had to certify that you had at least ten years of life left in order to get approval to conduct the operation," giving me even more confidence that I was beginning to put this issue into the background and could look forward to more active retirement years. Of course, that also made the doctor look like a "life saver."

Interestingly, I had NO pain. Yes, there was some discomfort in the groin and stomach area where they had conducted the procedure and made the slits in my body, but no pain. I confirmed with the doctor that I was being given the anti-inflammatory medicine, but I was receiving just a modest liquid dose of Tylenol. In fact, when I left the hospital, the prescription I had for Tylenol was for 325 mg tablets while the over-the-counter bottle included 500 mg in each pill. So, I dropped the prescription and decided to use the Tylenol pills I had if needed. And pain was never an issue. I attribute this to two factors: 1) the robotic surgery indeed is quite effective and dramatically reduces tissue trauma, and 2) my body fortunately has a high pain tolerance, which is basically a function of genes. The combination literally eliminated for me any pain in this surgical journey. That made me a lucky man (recall my friend in Sarasota).

The nurses in my hospital room were terrific, both the afternoon and evening team. Each shift, both a nurse and a nurse practitioner provided my care, and they catered to my every need. They were knowledgeable, empathetic and careful. They stayed with me for the next 24 hours and I thanked each one for being a nurse. Yes, the doctor performs the surgery, and needs years of training to acquire the skills to do it, but then you are in the hands of nurses who provide hour by hour help for your stay in the hospital. Mine were skilled, from multiple backgrounds and did a fabulous job.

I was able to get up and walk around the entire floor at about 11 pm on the night of the surgery, with one of the evening nurses walking with me. I ultimately was able to walk on my own but a bit tentatively when I began. Initially, I had to figure how to get out of the bed without straining my lower stomach area, and the nurse provided guidance on those moves. I was able to walk all around the entire floor.

During the walk, she also told me that this was the floor where gunshot victims also were recovering. At that time Chicago, was having double digit gunshot victims every week. Knowing those victims were sharing my recovery floor probably was more than I needed to know, but it is a fact that this highly rated hospital in downtown Chicago not only provided the skilled kind of surgery I had just had, but also cared for many of the shooting victims on Chicago streets, who also need skilled medical treatments.

At one point, I removed my gown from covering my body in order to observe what I looked like. I had 7 bandaged sutures, one relatively long – the one through which they extracted the prostate. Most of my pubic hair was shaved off. A catheter had been inserted into my penis up to my bladder, to give the urethra, which had been cut in two and then stitched back together, time to heal free of any irritation caused by the elimination flow of acidic urine. The catheter was firmly taped in multiple places to my body – thankfully – as one doesn't want it easily dislodged. Actually, at the end of the catheter that is in the bladder, there is a small bubble that also helps keep the catheter in place, i.e., from slipping out. But one doesn't want that to be the only element that held it in place. The complex taping job gave me assurance that it would take a pretty sizeable tug for the catheter to be dislodged, something I very much did not want to happen. The other end of catheter was attached to a urine bag, which was going to be my friend until the catheter was removed, sometime in the next 10-14 days (of course I was hoping for 10 days, clearly as soon as possible). Overall it wasn't exactly a pleasant sight, but at least the surgery itself was now in my rearview mirror.

About 7 A.M. the morning after the operation, the urologist resident burst into my room trailed by about five additional and more novice, and mixed gender, residents, threw off my covers and gown, and showed everyone how one looked after prostatectomy surgery. Not exactly how I had always wanted to expose myself, but ..... That was a bit of surprise though the group didn't linger, and I was covered before I could even feel shock or embarrassment. It should be clear at this point that if you use a university-based medical program, you will be observed at multiple times in multiple states as the attendant doctors train the residents. For short time periods, you are a "specimen." Yes, generally your privacy is respected but residents can only learn by looking and doing. That is the reality of using a university affiliated medical group, which on the other hand usually has the most up-to-date knowledge and equipment.

Home after Surgery

Before I was discharged the afternoon of the day after the surgery, I was given a lesson by the day nurse in how to change the urine bag, which was continuously draining urine from the catheter. Those directions were pretty straight forward, and I was advised to change the bag when it got three-fourths or so full. I also was shown how to wash my penis with Hibiclens, an antiseptic/antimicrobial soap. I thought I had that process of washing down pat after 75 years of practice, but I did learn a couple of new techniques from the female nurse, and the importance of washing every morning and evening before I went to sleep.

My wife picked me up, we went to the car, and she drove me home. When I arrived in our apartment, I was exhausted, went right to the bed in the guest room and fell asleep for about two hours. I was stone-cold out for those two hours. It takes several days if not weeks to regain one's energy after major surgery.

Another aspect of the recovery process is eating the right diet – to facilitate easy bowel movements. Having a bowel movement with a catheter in you is no easy task. First, it is not easy just to sit down and have the catheter sticking out of your penis; you have to suspend yourself a bit above the toilet seat. And one does not want to have a difficult time having a bowel movement as any pressure exerted is felt by the area that has just experienced surgery trauma and also causes the catheter to slightly move in and out of the penis. I know, gory and intimate details but also important realities. So, I was advised to eat light, easy to digest meals and to take a stool softener pill every night. The fact is that elimination is one of the major hurdles in recovering from any operation. It is absolutely critical for ongoing bodily functions but not straightforward.

That night we had spaghetti and tomato sauce.

I slept like a log the first night, sleeping straight through for about 7 hours. I had hooked the urine bag to the side of a waste basket that I placed right beside my bed, so it was below my body as I slept on my back. This allowed the urine to easily flow through the catheter and down into the collection bag. When I woke up in the morning and looked down, I was amazed at the volume. Yes I had drunk several glasses of liquid the day and night before, and emptied the urine bag several times, but it seemed like there was substantially more than a quart – maybe even a half gallon – of urine in the bag (I later learned the bag was large enough so that I did not have to worry about its over flowing during the night). It seemed that my body eliminated large amounts of urine during the night while I slept.

So, on that first day after coming home from the hospital I went on a quest for the "adult underwear" that would absorb such a volume. ☹ Another unpleasant reality of prostate surgery is that most men lose control over urination and it takes several weeks if not months to regain control. In the meantime, one must wear protective underwear or underwear pads so that the urine loss is collected before it seeps into your clothes. Ugh. And after looking at what I thought was a gigantic volume of nightly urine, 1 thought I needed a super absorbent underpant, something that could absorb gallons to get me through the night.

My wife and I surfed the web and found just the right item, a maximum absorbent pant that came with an iron clad guarantee to protect one through the night. I ended up buying two cases of the item, and then after two-to three nights realized I didn't need them. Nevertheless, I was prepared for the worst and would be fully protected for the next six months. I ended up giving those items to our local food pantry, which also provided clothes and other items for people in need, most of whom in our diverse Edgewater Chicago neighborhood are seniors.

But back to the morning after I left the hospital. I got out of bed, went to the bathroom and emptied that voluminous urine bag. That went easily. Then it was on to my first bowel movement, which was no piece of cake. There I was suspended over the toilet seat, holding my bag of urine, sort of trembling, and trying to have a relaxed bowel movement. Are you kidding me? Try it yourself sometime! It was not easy. Remember you have this catheter sticking out of your penis so you can't just sit down. I immediately realized that I should rest the urine bag in a waste basket, which I dragged over to the toilet; that freed-up hand helped. But I was still in sort of a suspended state. Fortunately, the movement happened quite effortlessly, and all went well, and I had made it through the elimination process the first morning without any major problems.

By that time, however, I was exhausted, so I walked into the living room, sat down, and took a short nap, before I drank my morning Joe, and read the newspaper. Since I still was ferrying the urine bag – a task I would be doing so for the next 10-14 days – I needed a place to set it everywhere I sat. So, I needed a waste basket at every chair and sofa around the apartment so I could set the bag into it and not have it tilting and trying to yank the catheter out of me. Ouch. I quickly figured that out, rounded up the needed number of waste baskets, and placed them in all strategic spots.

After finishing the newspaper and eating a modest breakfast, I decided to have a shower and get dressed. That also required some new agile moves. First, I had to figure out what to do with the urine bag while I was in the shower – remember it is attached to me every second until the catheter is extracted. Luckily, I had a grab bar in the shower, but it was at waist height so I couldn't hook the urine bag onto it. I needed the bag to be at least at knee level – below the bladder. So, I found some string and created a loop around the grab bar. I was able to hook the urine bag on the bottom portion of that loop after I stepped into the shower. Whew! I was making progress step by step. And then I showered, being careful not to slip and to be cautious down in the area of the slits, sutures and bandages. I also used the microbiological soap and cleaned my privates. I dried and then applied salve to the tip of the penis where the catheter was inserted, as that part can get quite tender.

Now, what could I wear? I couldn't just put on a pair of pants on and buckle up. My mid-section was still quite sensitive. Eleanor had purchased a pair of over-sized shorts for me, the next size up from my normal waist, and with a tie string. To get them on, I first had to thread the urine bag down through the legs, grab it when it had exited from the bottom of the leg, and then hoist up the shorts and tie them loosely around my midsection. I put on a golf shirt, walked to the living room, sat down and took another nap.

All I could think of was that I wanted the catheter out as soon as bloody possible. At some point in the first week home, the nurse called and said I was scheduled for removal of the catheter on a date, that was just 10 days from the surgery. Whoopee. I was elated. At least I didn't have to wait the entire two weeks.

Unexpected Phenomenon
During this wait, I had two other experiences about which I had not been forewarned, both of which were upsetting. First, I noted that there was some "dark solid stuff" in the urine bag, which looked like black pieces of skin. Not knowing what that was, I thought the urethra sutures were failing and that I'd have to go back into surgery and get them fixed. Second, often when I was in the midst of a bowel movement, when there was some

exertion to make it happen, a small amount of blood exited from the end of the penis. This also worried me.

So, I called the urologist's nurse, who usually called me back relatively quickly, always by the end of the day. She assured me that these were ordinary occurrences – the "dark stuff" was actually "tissue" from where the urethra had been cut – and not to worry. She also said the blood drops were common and would stop sometime soon, but to call if they expanded in number. And I did stop worrying, but I did see tissue several times the next two weeks as well as small drops of blood. Over time both stopped.

Finally, the time came for the catheter to be removed. THANK GOD. We arrived at the doctor's office a few minutes early and were ushered into a patient room almost immediately. The nurse arrived, took off all the tape keeping the catheter tethered to my body, somehow burst the bubble that was at the end of the catheter, and then asked me to breathe out heavily while she quickly removed the tube. It stung a bit as she yanked it out, but it was out. WHEW! I thanked her profusely. And she smiled, knowing this procedure made me very happy. She gave me what looked like an adult "huggie" and said that would protect me now that the catheter was gone.

She said guys never missed this appointment. In fact, she said that the previous January three guys were scheduled to have the catheter removed on a day when there was a terrific snowstorm in Chicago. Most people did not go to work, and schools were closed. Nevertheless, she said with a smile,

"All three men made it on time and not a one missed the appointment!"

She then said that in a month they would take my PSA. The hope was that it would be zero, but she also said it should at least be below 1 and could be in the low one-hundredths, like maybe 0.15 and maybe even lower than that. And that the expectation was that it would gradually decline to a low number, at least below 0.05. Further, she said, that they would watch the PSA for the next several months expecting it to drop gradually, and ideally to zero. More on this below.

Informing Loved Ones and Friends

At about this time, I sent an email to my family members and other friends, the intent of which was both to inform them of my situation but also to encourage all the men to continue to get PSA tests and if they had elevated PSAs that the doctor wanted to diagnose further, to ask for MRIs before any biopsy. Here is what I wrote:

> I am writing to give you an update on my health situation, having had surgery to remove my prostate on June 5. Some of you knew this was going to happen and others did not, so I'm giving everyone the whole story here.
>
> Even though I am over 70, I was getting my PSA test every year, and while flat until I was 70, it began creeping up in 2015. Last summer it got to just over 7. My internist said it was time to see the urologist. The subsequent diagnosis process and then treatment was different from what I had expected.
>
> The urologist said he wouldn't rush anything. The first step was what he called an enhanced PSA test, to see if the rise in the PSA was due to free antigens, which was a good thing, or antigens probably linked to cancer. I had virtually no free antigens.
>
> The next step was an MRI of the prostate; it showed I had two and possibly three lesions (cancer areas). That led to a biopsy, but a biopsy targeted to those three areas, plus a few additional random areas.
>
> The results came back. The medical team gave each biopsy two scores on a scale of 1-5. These

two numbers are added to provide a Gleason core. The two suspect lesions had a Gleason score of 3+4, or 7. Anything 6 or less puts you in the "watchful waiting" category. Anything 8 or above puts you in the "do something now" category. My scores were in the transition area. But any sub-score of 4 or 5 is dangerous, with a 4 being intermediate risk and a 5 being major risk.

The doc said nothing much would change over the winter so I should go ahead and spend the winter in Florida, which I did. My treatment options were basically surgery or radiation (40 zaps, 5 times a week over an 8-week period, which I opted against—the major error is zapping the colon which I did not want).

When I got back to Chicago from Florida, I had the surgery on June 5. I was wheeled into the OR at 7:30 and got to the recovery room at 11:00 am. The surgery is laparoscopic and robotic; you get six small slits across your groin area and another above the belly button through which the surgeons insert the robots and use one to extract the prostate. The surgeons sit at a large console, which magnifies things about ten times, manipulating the robots and what they do. I had the main surgeon, and then about 5 residents as the Northwestern Urology Department is well known for this procedure.

Everything went well; I was home by 3:30 the next day walking around. The catheter was removed a week later on Tuesday, June 12; the nurse said guys never miss that appointment, even when there is a major snowstorm! And now it is just a matter of getting bladder control again, and I'm happy with the progress I am making.

The post-op pathology report found Gleason scores of 4+3, or 7s, now with the dominant score the 4. So, it was a good thing I took action. But during the operation they saw no sign of spread and did not need to do anything with the lymph nodes. They will continue to take my PSA every three months for the next two years, just to make sure nothing remains, but the docs are pleased with what they found and what they did.

Given all the false positives one hears about with the PSA, I was pleased to see the new steps during the diagnosis process and the targeted biopsy after the MRI; just a few years ago I had friends who had 14 random biopsies with no MRI directing those procedures. And the robotic surgery is quite amazing; I had virtually no pain; yes, some discomfort sitting down and rising up but no pain. My pain prescription med was 325 mg Tylenol! Less than is in one Tylenol PM pill.

The two major risks for these treatments are incontinence and impotence, both of which are nasty, but in my mind better than prostate cancer, which leads to a painful death.

It's going to take me 4-6 weeks to fully recover and get back to my golf game, but now I will have another excuse for not shooting as well as I want!

One other thing. The doc said he could not do the operation unless he predicted I'd live another 10 years. Good news for me, and also a caution for those our age to not delay things so long until an operation is ruled out.

I received multiple responses to this email, many thanking me for the detail. Further, several men also ordered a PSA test during a subsequent physical, with many of those having doctors who had not been requiring the test.

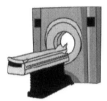

5

Regaining Bladder Control

Now that the catheter was out, I had the new challenges of what to do given that I did not have bladder control. ☹ The nurse first gave me a set of exercises to strengthen my "pelvic floor," i.e., to regain bladder control. These exercises are called "Kegels." You tighten, or squeeze together, your lower pelvic muscles as if you are trying to hold back gas or trying to stop the flow of urine. These exercises work to strengthen the sphincter muscles down there – those affecting both urine and stool.

The Kegel regime started at 10 quick squeezes, then 5 longer squeezes about 3 seconds each, and ended with ten short squeezes. I was supposed to do this for a week. In Week 2, I was to increase the short squeezes to 20 each, and the longer holds to 5 seconds each. In Week 3, the short squeezes were raised to 25, followed by five 7-second holds, and then 25 quick contractions. In week 4, the short contractions were raised to 30, and the five holds to 7 seconds. By week 5, which I was to continue until I regained bladder control, I was to do 30 quick contractions, 5 ten-second holds, and then another 30 quick contractions. And I was to do these exercises four times a day. Further, I was advised to follow the regime as specified because while I was working to strengthen the areas that had endured the trauma of surgery, I was not to overdo it, or I would actually not heal.

There were a couple of other exercises which I did mainly on the floor by raising my hips and doing the Kegel, again to strengthen my pelvic floor when my body got into unusual positions.

Kegel exercises and more turn out to be aspects of the solution for other medical problems among my age-cohort friends. One male friend wrote that he had serious urinary urgency problems (not related to prostate cancer) and was seeing a physical therapist, also a young, attractive female therapist, as it turns out. He needed to do Kegel exercise, which she called "elevator up," to strengthen his ability to not urinate, and another exercise, which she called "elevator down," sort of a "pushing" exercise, to enhance his ability to completely empty his bladder when he did urinate. Try doing that without farting or defecating! In a "hands on" approach to assessing how my friend was doing in this aspect of his groin area, she monitored his exercises by inserting her (gloved) fingers into his rectum to make sure he was moving the right muscles. Just another example of what older males might face as issues in their groin areas atrophy with old age.

Finally, the nurse said I should take a Viagra pill every other day to get "blood flowing into that area of the body," knowing I knew which area she was referencing. Ok, that is cool. BUT at $60 a pop that would be $900 a month. OMG, I was going to go broke. At my one-month-after surgery appointment, however, the doctor reduced this medication to twice a week, but still that was $480 a month. So, when I arrived in Florida, I found a place where one could order such meds from Canada or New Zealand at a cost of $7 a pill. (I also asked some friends whether they had the same erectile condition I had and asked them where they purchased their meds and was given several recommendations of web sites. I had to approach these queries a bit indirectly as no one had previously been bragging about being engaged in such commerce!)

I was about to leave when the nurse also suggested I do a Kegel when I got into and out of the car, and when I sat in or got up from a chair, sofa or toilet seat. Each time that action happens, she said, a strain is put on your pelvic floor and, given my weak muscles down there, without a held Kegel, the result would be a spurt of urine. That made me think maybe the catheter and urine bag weren't so bad an idea after all!

We left the office and found our car in the parking garage. I sat down without doing a Kegel and felt the spurt. OMG, this was going to get old really quickly. But I had been warned. Eleanor drove us home.

I was feeling pretty good and asked her to let me off on Bryn Mawr so I could walk a few blocks. She looked at me like I was nuts, but I said I felt pretty good. Confidently, I walked a few blocks but then fatigue swept over me and I turned back to home. I walked through the front door and beat a path to my bed in the guest bedroom and fell into a deep sleep for two solid hours. (Just to make the point, I had not been kicked out of our bedroom, but I did need access to several medical supplies and the guest bed was much closer to the toilet in the guest room and, given my condition, it simply was easier for me to use the guest bed. After a couple of weeks, I moved back to our king size bed in the master bedroom.)

Man Pads

When I woke up, now without the catheter and urine bag, I had to figure out what to do about my leaking bladder. All you are told is that there will be some incontinence after prostate surgery. Fine, but what does that mean? Spurts? How voluminous? Continual leakage? Dribbles? How much leakage, etc.? Could I feel it? I was quite uninformed. I did have two cases of the super absorbent adult huggies, but was wearing that every day and all day and night long my fate now? I really didn't know.

So, for the rest of the day, I wore what the nurse had given me. And it worked. At night, I donned the super absorbent adult huggie (that is not the official name, but it was how my mind viewed it). When I woke up, I thought I'd be soaked, but I wasn't. If fact, not much urine had leaked out during the night. Wow, that was nice. And that was an omen for my night experiences. I really didn't leak much at night (even though with the catheter I was draining out what seemed like quarts.).

The next day, therefore, I decided to go to the neighborhood drug store to see what the options were for handling the leakage. My first thought was to put a bag over my head so no one would recognize me; I had always avoided the adult underwear aisle and really didn't want to meet anyone I knew while there. But then I decided that thought that was silly. But I also thought I could go to a store far from where I lived to guarantee I could conduct this mission in secret. But then thought that was also silly. So, I sucked it up once again (my ab muscles were actually strengthening from all the sucking up I had done during this journey) and told myself,

"You can handle this. Be a man and just march in there like you know what you are doing," which I did.

The problem was I didn't know what I was doing. I knew there were going to be some technical issues; every now and then I had walked down the feminine hygiene aisle in the grocery store and saw words like heavy and light flow, maximum absorbent, pads, napkins, etc. and I figured I now was going to get a male version of this. Which indeed was the case. I walked through the door of the local drug store and sauntered, in what I thought was a casual manner, over to the adult underwear aisle. There was a women's and men's section. I stopped in front of the men's section, trying to look like an analytic scholar. Now what did I need: the full Depends version of the adult huggie, and if so, with the regular or the "fitted leg" opening, or just pads? But then, which pads – the one for "drips and dribbles" or the one for "larger spurts?" God, this wasn't easy. And I really didn't know. So, I bought a box of each!

Over a couple of weeks, I did figure it out what I needed. After wearing the super absorbent adult "huggie" (of which I had two cases) for several nights and noting that I was not leaking that much at night, I switched to the Depends fitted leg version, which was less bulky. Over time, I switched again first to the "larger spurts" pad, then to the "drips and dribbles" pad and finally and within several weeks to nothing at night. Similarly, I started wearing the full Depends pant during the day, but soon learned I didn't need it; without the catheter I was not leaking a steady stream. It was some combination of spurts and dribbles, spurts when I forgot to do a Kegel when sitting down or getting up or putting stress on my pelvic area such as when I lifted something, and pretty much drips and dribbles the other time. Ultimately, I "graduated" to just the drips and dribbles pad, which I discovered was not that big a deal to wear.

I did have to change my underwear approach. I had been wearing "boxers," but they are not amenable to accommodating pads. So, I had to switch to briefs, but to jazz it up a bit, I bought colored briefs and not the old but standard "tighty whities."

I apologize sharing all these leaky details but at the time they were a big deal, and I had no knowledge of what to expect. I hope this foray into urine incontinence and adult underwear items is helpful to the reader.

Of course, the BIG question was how long all this would last? When would I regain bladder control? The doctor and nurse said about 3-6 months. I was hoping for the shorter rather than the longer time period. At about this time, I also discovered other relatives and friends who had gone through this process. And I talked with each one of them, asking about this issue. Unfortunately, they all had their prostate removed when they were much younger than I, and their younger and stronger pelvic muscles enabled them to restore bladder control in a matter of weeks. I was 75, several weeks into recovery and still having leakage.

Actually, I did not have much leakage, except when I went on my daily 4-mile walk. So regaining bladder control focused in a relatively short time period on getting it for the long walk. When I was home and just moving around the apartment – or house when we had returned to Sarasota – there was no leakage. At one point the nurse said that another exercise to strengthen your pelvic sphincter muscles was to ride a bike, which I did when we arrived in Sarasota, and that pretty much did the trick – solved the leakage issue. Although I could still have modest leakage for the next several months, when my body got into an unusual position like lifting something or turning and still sometimes when I took a long walk, it was intermittent. I pretty much became leakage free. And I continued to do the Kegel exercises every day.

Incidentally, my other brother who informed me of his stage 4 esophageal cancer the weekend before my prostate surgery died two weeks after talking to me; he never lived the 3-6 months his doctor had given him.

Luckily, the celebration of life service was held in mid-July of 2018 and by then I was healed enough from the prostatectomy and able to travel and be there for the service.

Cancer Recurrence

Of course, while bladder control was an issue, it was not a matter of life and death. Getting rid of the cancer was. I was most interested in my PSA level.

When I returned for my one-month check-up, I got a bit of a shock. The doctor said that the pathology report on the prostate found that microscopic amounts of cancer, not visible to the naked eye, had actually escaped the prostate sac around the area of the bulge! He felt the probability was that nothing remained in my body and that the bad guys that had managed to escape the prostate probably remained on the prostate, which had been removed. But it was clear that some could have slithered down and remained in my body around the prostate area.

The nurse then drew blood for my first post-surgery PSA test. After successful treatment of the prostate (either removal via surgery or demolition via radiation), the PSA count is supposed to drop to zero or a negligible number, like <0.05. Mine didn't. This test showed that my PSA dropped, but only to 0.12. The doctor and nurse said not to worry and to hope/expect it would continue to drop. They further said that at the one-month period the PSA often does not drop to zero. At that appointment, the doctor further noted that his standard for concern was a PSA of 0.1 or less, that if the PSA didn't stay at or below that level, additional treatment might be required. After the appointment, I immediately went on the web, where most articles posited a standard of 0.2, and I was well below that. But the articles also said that a substantial rise, particularly a doubling of the PSA count, would indicate trouble.

Two months later in September, when I had my annual physical – annual wellness – visit with my internist, another blood sample was drawn and the PSA had dropped further to 0.10, a good sign –still not zero, but it was moving in the right direction. The weird element here was that I got the results via an electronic medical record system, which noted that my PSA was in the "normal range," at this point a phrase that was meaningless for my situation. Mine should be just about zero and the electronic message should be revised for a man who had had prostate cancer surgery.

A month later in October, when I had my four-month after-surgery visit with my urologist/surgeon, the nurse again took a blood sample. I was hoping the PSA would decline another notch. But it did not: the PSA had risen to 0.11 just modestly above my doctor's standard but still below the 0.2 web standard. The doctor mulled this and then said,

"Let's give it another couple of months and hope it resumes a downward trek."

A technical comment. PSA measures to the hundredth decimal place and to below 1.0 are a relatively recent phenomenon. Ten or so years ago the technology was not sufficient to detect such specific and low counts; years ago, in this situation, I would have been told everything was fine, that my PSA was undetectable. But today the PSA tests are much more finely tuned and can detect counts below 1 and to the hundredths of a decimal point. In retrospect this was good for me, though at the time certainly gave me cause – good cause it turned out – to worry.

Nevertheless, my wife and I left Chicago for Sarasota a week later. I took with me an order to get a PSA test in two months. In early December, I went to one of the Quest Diagnostics Labs in Sarasota which drew a blood test and sent it out for a PSA count analysis; the result, which was faxed to my Chicago urologist, was a PSA of 0.21. Disappointingly, my PSA was increasing, yes at a low level, but it was rising and now had doubled. My nurse in Chicago said the high result could be due to how that lab worked perhaps differently from the one at Northwestern Memorial Hospital where all the other PSA analyses had been conducted. I said we'd be in Chicago for New Year's Eve and she said to get a PSA test in the Northwestern Memorial lab when I arrived. I did.

I got the results from the nurse who called me at 4 pm on New Year's Eve: PSA count of 0.21.

She said in a sympathetic tone, "You need to see the radiation oncologist."

What a message to receive on the cusp of New Year's Eve. I was shaking. Everything had gone well with the surgery, and I was fully recovered, meaning I had regained control over my bladder functions. But the cancer was still inside me. Had I gone through all the agony of the surgery just to be back where I started? Would I make it through this second treatment phase? Would I die before I thought I would? And I dreaded radiation, which I knew was a Monday through Friday event for eight weeks, and with possible unpleasant side effects. I was bummed.

More Friendly Advice

I sent an email notice to several friends of my new situation. The following supportive response helped prepare for me this next stage in my journey:

> *Oh, Allan, I'm sorry to learn of your new prostate developments. Like I said, there is never 100% certainty that we are done with any of the messy stuff of life and health, like cancer.*
>
> *Ten years ago, my PSA remained measurable and increased after my (botched) prostatectomy. Metastasis was assumed, even though a full body scan did not find anything suspicious. And so, I was referred to the head oncologist at the Mayo Clinic. He first gave me the opportunity to sign up*

for a clinical trial but then, at the last minute, called me back to Mayo for an MRI, which solved the mystery: the surgery had removed only part of my prostate. (That clinical trial, by the way, seemed promising — a shot to super-boost one's immune system — but it later proved to be ineffective.) So, I had a successful salvage surgery and slowly got back to somewhat normal life — until the tiny increases in PSA brought me to a second go-round this past year...

Regarding hormone therapy, this is what I think I know: The shot of Lupron, administered in the buttocks, doesn't hurt but is powerful. I took a daily pill (Casodex) the first few weeks, because Lupron actually boosts testosterone initially, before it effectively shuts down production of the male hormone. The main side effect, hot flashes, did not kick in for me until a few months later. The side effects of weight gain and bone/muscle loss are less obvious but real. I continued to exercise as much as I could.

Four months after the androgen deprivation – Lupron – shot, I moved into Hope Lodge at the Mayo Clinic in Rochester, Minnesota, and began my 38 daily radiation treatments (of two centiGreys each). This is when a strong dose of daily supplements was recommended by my radiation oncologist and his nurse/assistant, as follows: 1) Calcium Magnesium Citrate (600mg) — two in the morning, two late in the day; 2) Magnesium (400mg) — one/day, 3) Vitamin D3 (2,000 IU) — one/day, 4) A small heated glassful of water with EmergenC (1/2 package) with Collagen (Type 1 & 3, 6600 mg).

In addition and more randomly, I also took various substances said to aide with side-effects: fish oil, Move Matrix (Type 2 Collagen), Miso - fermented soybean paste - (spoonful/day, to counteract bad effects of radiation, a food that my wife consumes every day, but that I didn't like at all, even mixed with peanut butter!). [This was on top of my few regular Rxs (Occuvite, for eye health) and Levothyroxine (low dose thyroid med), plus the occasional Andrographis Paniculata at first sign of a cold. I felt like a pill-pusher!]

An amusing side story: During my last half-marathon ski race before moving to Rochester last March, I met another Mayo radiation oncologist who had traveled all the way to our neck of the woods to ski a short 8K race. I thought him an odd fellow because he couldn't stop recommending that I follow up my radiation with daily doses of ginseng (not just any ginseng, but Wisconsin ginseng). Apparently, a Mayo double-blind study demonstrated its effectiveness in combating post-radiation exhaustion. My own radiation oncologist was not particularly impressed with the study. It turned out that a good Ely friend who had been at Mayo for CA treatments had purchased two bottles of the recommended WI Ginseng but was unable to use them for some reason and so gifted me with them; upon returning home I dutifully took several pills daily until they were gone — but had no way of knowing if it did any good...

The hot flashes became fairly frequent and well-defined. Several times a night I would need to throw off the covers and sometimes change my sweaty t-shirt. Several months after my "six-month" shot, the hot flashes gradually became less frequent, less well-defined, less intense — and now, 14 months after my shot, they are history.

Another definite side-effect of my therapies: the need for more sleep. I always slept up to eight hours a night, and often also took a brief after-lunch nap. Since my hormone and radiation *therapies began, I've slept nine or ten hours a night and some days take two short naps!*

Well, I hope my experience is of some help/comfort. Best wishes for outcome of your scans! Keep in touch.

E.B., Minnesota

This note was exceedingly comforting, as I had NO idea of what would happen in the next phase of treatments, but now I had a good overview of the experience of a friend my age.

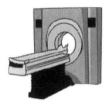

6

Radiation and Hormone Therapy

We had a flight back to Sarasota on January 4th and luckily were able to schedule an appointment with the radiation oncologist, on January 3rd, the day before we left. Right after I got the word from the urologist's nurse that I should see the radiation oncologist, I dialed the number for his office (remember, this was late afternoon on New Year's Eve). A voice answered and I responded that I'd like to schedule an appointment with the radiation oncologist next week, before the 4th. He said the doctor was booked but would give me the number of the nurse who controlled his detailed schedule. I thanked him and called that nurse. Luckily, she also was still in the office. I explained my situation and she squeezed me in on the third.

Meeting the Radiation Oncologist

We arrived a bit early for our appointment with the radiation oncologist. The radiation oncology offices are in the lower concourse, the name Northwestern Memorial Hospital gives to what us normal folks call the basement. Maybe running a radiation beam all day long is actually best done in the basement. As long as the beam points down, it can't accidentally hit anything or one on any lower floor! Whatever. The office complex was quite nice and there were several people, mostly men, in the check-in area waiting to get their daily zap. Most looked calm.

We were ushered into a patient room within one or two minutes of our appointment time. One goal of the hospital is to have patient's wait time be as short as possible. The resident oncologist arrived first. He asked me to review my history, as he followed along both taking notes and reading from papers he had, which I assume had the history. He said it was good that we were considering this option now as that put us ahead of the curve in terms of treating the recurrence. He further said that the lead radiation oncologist had decades of experience and high levels of success with his patients. That was assuring. He then said the doctor would probably recommend both hormone therapy, which would start before the radiation therapy, and radiation therapy, with the former occurring for probably a year or two! That was a surprise; no one – except my friend – previously had mentioned that I'd get a double dose of treatments at this next step, but my wife and I just listened. He said they probably would first do a bone scan as well as additional MRIs of my abdomen and prostate area.

A bone scan! Yikes. When prostate cancer spreads, it goes onto and then into the bones and if it does the latter, then it is at stage four and there is no cure. So, my heart began beating a bit – actually a lot – faster. He said there was minimal – pretty much negligible – chance that these tests would show anything, but they were standard diagnostics before the next stage of therapies would begin.

The radiation oncologist then arrived. He had a complicated last name, so everyone called him Dr. John. He reiterated what the resident had just said. He also said prostate cancer moves slowly – very slowly – and we were catching the recurrence very early so the prognosis for success was excellent. He further said he would recommend hormone therapy as well as radiation therapy. The hormone therapy would starve the remaining cancer cells and if it did not "off" (my word) the cancer still in my body, the radiation would "kill" (his word) whatever remained. He then said that before they would launch the treatments, I needed a bone scan and MRI of my abdomen and pelvic area. He finished by saying that if the scan and MRIs were negative, which he fully expected, he would start the hormone therapy right away, followed after about two months with the radiation treatment, which would indeed be the 8-week regimen with radiation zaps (my word) Monday through Friday. He said there would be few side effects of these treatments, the most common being hot flashes from the hormone treatment and possibly diarrhea from the radiation, and that I likely would be quite fatigued by the end of the radiation treatment.

I then asked him, "How tired?", as my wife and I had planned a three-week trip in July to Bordeaux, Paris, a river cruise to Normandy for the 75th anniversary of D-Day, and then a few days in London.

He said, "You'll be fine by then, perhaps a bit more tired than usual, but you will fully be able to enjoy such a trip and the river cruise."

He concluded by saying, "Don't postpone the trip; take the trip."

That was that. I was in somewhat of a state of shock, both hearing that I'd be getting two treatments and being a bit nervous that while a negligible probability of finding anything, they would conduct a bone scan as well as MRIs of my lower body to see if any of my cancer had spread. And that my second round of treatments would be backing up to the beginning of our trip to France and England. Oh well, it is what it is, and it was good that we were catching this recurrence early.

We were escorted to his scheduling nurse and the doctor asked her to schedule me for the scans and the MRIs. I asked if they could somehow squeeze me in the next week, so I could delay my return to Sarasota, but that was not possible. The appointments were made for Monday, January 21, with a follow up at 7 A.M. on Wednesday, January 23, which would allow me to make an 11 A.M. flight that day back to Sarasota. I wanted to continue playing golf and duplicate bridge!

We had dinner that night with some good friends. One of the questions they asked was if I was going to get a second opinion. I had not thought about that as I had confidence in the urology and oncology departments in the Northwestern Memorial medical group. But the friend suggested I call a mutual doctor friend, who also worked at Northwestern.

The next day I did just that. He said my situation was not unusual, and that the standard protocol these days was the combined hormone and radiation therapies. He shared an example of another person he had known, who lived in a more rural area, and encountered the same prostate recurrence that I had, and whose doctor had recommended hormone and radiation. That person then paid on his own for a second opinion from the Mayo Clinic in Rochester, Minnesota, where those doctors suggested the identical treatment. He said my condition was common and the proposed treatment my oncologist had recommended was now standard practice in the medical community and that I had well known and experienced doctors at Northwestern – so there was no real need for a second opinion. He also said that radiation treatment today is much more precise than it was ten years ago, minimizing the possibility of an accidental zapping of my colon. He said those mistakes rarely happen these days. All this information was comforting.

A couple days later, after I had sent out a short email to many friends concerning my prostate cancer recurrence and the upcoming hormone and radiation therapies, I had a long conversation with a close doctor friend of mine in Madison. He also said my situation was common and that I was going to receive what the field considered the standard therapies – both hormone and radiation therapies. He said those treatments were highly effective. He even used the word "curative." His comments were also very soothing, coming from a close and knowledgeable friend.

I also went on the web and found similar results in articles on recurrent prostate cancer in the National Institutes of Health's website. This website had even more information. Both therapies individually were effective, and the combination was even more effective. Actually, the medical literature did not use the word "effective" for these treatments, but used the phrase "five-year survival rate," gulp. I'd actually prefer to see a ten-year survival rate, if you follow my drift, but all that was provided for my situation was the five-year survival rate. For hormone therapy alone for recurrent prostate cancer, the five-year survival rate was about 95 percent. For radiation therapy alone for recurrent prostate cancer, the five-year survival rate also was about 95 percent. For the combined therapies together for recurrent prostate cancer, the five-year survival rate was "virtually 100 percent." That sounded pretty good. That would get me to 81! And after that, I wasn't going to have that many more five-year periods of life anyway!

Planning for Hormone and Radiation Therapy

I returned to Chicago on January 20 for my diagnostic tests the next day. Everything went on schedule.

A bone scan is a nuclear medicine test that helps physicians diagnose and track several types of bone disease, in my case metastasized prostate cancer. The whole-body bone scan was conducted in two parts. Upon arrival, the nurse inserted an intravenous (IV) line into a vein in my arm; as noted in a previous chapter, this took some effort – about three tries before the IV was firmly in place. She then injected a radioactive tracer into the IV. It took several hours for my bloodstream to carry the tracer to all bones in my body.

So, after the getting the internal tracer into my blood stream but before the actual bone scan, I went to the MRI lab where I got the MRIs, the abdomen one that covered the liver, kidney and lower intestines, and the pelvic one that covered the prostate area. Then I returned and had the bone scan.

When I returned for the bone scan, it took approximately 35 minutes to complete that test. During the test, I lay flat on a table. Multiple images of my anatomy were taken, at timed intervals, using a nuclear medicine camera. The images were then reviewed by a radiologist and a report sent to my ordering physician – my oncologist – after 48 hours.

I returned to the radiation oncologists office at 7 A.M. Wednesday morning and got the results – everything, as expected but now confirmed, was negative. There were no visible signs of metastasized prostate cancer. Wonderful! Now on to the treatments.

The hormone therapy consists of two parts; there is a pill – my doctor prescribed Bicalutamide -- and then a Lupron shot that is administered once every four months. I had also read about both of these on the web. The objective of hormone therapy is to reduce if not eliminate testosterone, an androgen hormone, as prostate cancer lives off androgens – hormones that produce masculine characteristics, testosterone being a major one. The hormone therapy is designed to kill the cancer via starvation. While the Lupron is quite powerful in reducing the body's testosterone production, it initially induces the body to make more testosterone, the opposite of what is wanted. The Bicalutamide pill offsets that tendency, so the two work in concert – the pill actually offsetting those initial tendencies of the Lupron.

I was given a prescription for the Bicalutamide and said I'd fill it in Sarasota. The glitch was that I needed to take the Bicalutamide pills at least for two weeks before getting the Lupron shot. So, if I was in Sarasota, I'd need to get the Lupron shot there. That shot was quite expensive – and part of a complex treatment protocol. Though I tried to find a urologist in Sarasota to give the shot (this shot is given by the urologist and not the radiation oncologist by the way), none were willing to do so unless I shifted my treatment regimen over to their office, which I was not willing to do. It also turned out to be impossible for the Northwestern group to order the shot for me to pick up at a drug store. After a couple of frustrating days, I phoned my favorite nurse at my urologist's office and scheduled an appointment to get the shot in Chicago at 8:30 A.M. on February 8. It would entail an extra trip to Chicago but now my Chicago medical team would be in charge of all my treatments.

I got the papers outlining what I was to do for the radiation prep appointment and was told to return to the oncologist offices on April 3.

I started the hormone pills when I returned to Sarasota. Two weeks later, after playing duplicate bridge on Thursday afternoon, February 7, I drove to Tampa to catch a flight to Chicago that evening. After a short night's sleep, I hopped out of bed, took the bus downtown to the Northwestern Hospital, walked into the urologists' office at 8:28, was ushered into the patient room right away, dropped my pants and got my first Lupron shot in my right butt.

I didn't know exactly how long the doctor would keep me on this therapy, but I made an appointment in June to have the second Lupron booster shot. I was now fully into the hormone therapy.

I returned to Sarasota that day, and resumed my activities there – golfing, duplicate bridge, cooking, gardening, etc. My wife and I also started ballroom dancing lessons. I was having fun and so far, had no side effects from the hormone therapy. I lived the next two months as if I had no cancer but hoping the hormone therapy was working to starve the cancer cells still in my body. The time quickly arrived for me to return to Chicago.

Starting Hormone Therapy and Preparing for Radiation

I left Sarasota in late March and drove to Chicago. My appointment to begin the radiation treatment was scheduled for the following Wednesday, April 3rd. I encouraged Eleanor to remain in Florida as the good, 80-degree weather was just arriving and I would not begin the actual radiation treatment, when she wanted to be near to provide support, until April 10 (which then was extended to the 17th).

Initially, I had quite limited knowledge about how the hormone therapy would impact me over time, nor did I know much about the process of the radiation therapy. At first, I thought these both would be a slam-dunk but now that I was getting into the middle of it, I admitted it posed significant challenges to the male persona.

Let me elaborate.

First, hormone therapy reduces the body's testosterone, which already is pretty low for a 76-year-old male. Basically, it eliminates what little is left at my age. The side effects are: weight gain, fatigue, low libido, hot flashes, breast enlargement, genital shrinkage, etc. Cool, huh? The latter two came as somewhat of a surprise (docs don't always tell you everything, although what man hasn't said at one time or another, I'd give my left nut for _____? so now I was going to shrink both "nuts" as well as the main member to save my life, not a bargain I had anticipated but one I now had to make!). Lucky me.

And hot flashes – they began on April Fool's Day, the Monday after I had returned to Chicago. Like my friend, I had none the first two months I was on hormone therapy. Initially, I thought the possibility of hot flashes was a joke, as I wasn't having any. But as I sat watching the news on Monday, April 1 and my body got hotter and hotter, I suddenly realized, OMG, the hot flashes are here. And even though it was April Fools, they were no joke! They began to come and go several times a day; the experience could be worse, but it was helping me handle the cold Chicago spring, so I guess there was some upside to this side-effect. And I received no sympathy for this new phenomenon when I told Eleanor, and other women friends; they all just chuckled and said, "Welcome to my world."

And then, on April 3, I went to the doctor's office to prep for the radiation therapy itself. For the uninitiated, radiation is when they shoot a beam into your groin area to kill any remaining prostate cells. Actually, radiation interferes with the process of cells regenerating themselves. Further, radiation impacts both healthy cells and cancer cells that are in the radiated area. The healthy tissue that is damaged by the radiation is able to cure itself through cell regeneration; the cancer cells are not able to regenerate after radiation so are killed in the process.

The beam is powerful and destroys its target. Of course, the groin is a pretty sensitive area, where one doesn't want anyone to make a mistake! Who knows what will be singed if the beam is off by just a bit? You get my drift?

I said to the nurse who was poking around down there,

"How does the radiation beam actually work.?"

She said, "The beam encircles the entire prostate area and sometimes could hit the urethra [and you know where that is] so if you have any burning sensation when you urinate, please tell me."

Of course, that made me think what else might get burned or singed ☹ during radiation and when was the last time you told a female you did not know that you had a burning sensation in your penis when urinating? I soon learned that this was just the beginning of confiding all sorts of intimate experiences with young nurses, gulpl

To get set up for the radiation, I went to the (un)dressing room to take off my pants and underwear and put on a gown, which must have been a mini gown because it hit someplace on my thigh several inches above my knee. Then I walked into the CT Sim room where two nurses awaited me. Wow. And all I had covering my private parts was that flimsy (and short) gown ☹.

Then I thought, OMG, I knew that with my testosterone virtually eliminated spontaneous erections were few and far between, but what if it happened here? Gulp! Oh, please God, make my body behave. So, I tugged my mini-gown down a bit, putting my hand in front of my you know what.

And then one of the nurses said, "Go ahead, and lie on the table."

OMG, again, would the gown be long enough to continue to cover me or would I be laying there flashing those two?" Fortunately, the other nurse asked if I'd like a warm blanket on me?

I said, actually almost shouted, "Yes."

So, while the one nurse stood behind me and deftly raised my gown a bit, the other skillfully put the warm blanket over my mid-section. Phew, I became fully covered.

Instantaneously, both of them started poking around down there adjusting the blanket so that it exposed all my short hairs (I guess in order to get a better X-ray) but ended right at the beginning of you know what. Once again, I said a prayer that Mr. Wonderful would realize this was a medical procedure and just lie there relaxed, like I was (Ha!), but you have to admit it all was becoming a bit tricky. Actually, I was thinking this was akin to what Robert Craft (owner of the Patriots for those uninformed) is alleged to have experienced at that Florida massage parlor just south of in Orlando!

Then they did the scan and I thought everything was over. But no. Now both came over to me, moved that blanket down even further, exposing more short hairs and just the beginning of you know what, and began to make the spots that would guide my placement on the radiation table so the Radiation Beam would hit just the right spots. Oh man, I thought, "Please do this fast and let me stay relaxed." When the two had finally marked everything with a magic marker, I thought once again I was done, but no!

One of the nurses came over and said, "Now I have to give you three tattoos which cannot be washed off."

Tattoos? Wow, that's cool. Would I get roses or a heart or arrows or what, and what colors could I choose, and were there any choices? Actually, no choices, and the tats were just larger black dots. ☹ The tats on my sides went just fine but she had to work a bit harder to put one just at the beginning of my you know what. By that time, I was sweating a bit, and wondering if I was getting another hot flash. Finally, she said we were done, and to go get dressed and wait outside the dressing room, which I did.

Then a fourth nurse bounced around the corner and said come with me. She had the "educational" part of this beginning procedure, where you talk about urinating, urine stream strength, bowel movement, stool size, and other interesting aspects of what those parts of your body do on a daily basis.

One friend told me that at this stage, he actually was asked to drop his trousers and urinate into a container so the nurse would witness his "urinary stream strength." I was glad that hadn't been my experience!

Of course, talking to the nurse about all these issues was a novel experience because I hadn't had that many detailed conversations about those issues with my wife, let alone a person whom I'd just met. But I sucked it up (once again strengthening my abs) and engaged the conversation.

She began by saying that burning sensations when I urinate were possible as the therapy progressed. She looked up and asked if I knew what that was, and said, "You know, sometimes when you wake up in the morning and have to go really badly, often there is a momentary burning sensation?"

And I said, "Oh, yes, that has happened."

But then I asked, "Why should that happen as they would be radiating my prostate area, not the entire member, I mean area."

And she said, "Well, you know the prostate surrounds the urethra, and you know where the urethra is, and that entire area needs to be radiated so at times the beam could hit the urethra (ignoring what other organ it would need to pass through to do that)."

At that point, I just said, "Yes," and waved her on.

She then said. "You also need to go on a 'low residue' diet."

I blinked looking at her with questioning eyes that asked, "What is that?"

She said that means a diet with very little fiber, as the goal for the radiation was to have as clear a colon as possible.

And then I said. "Gee, I've been told for years to eat lots of fiber, in order to be regular, which would then clear my bowel so it would be perfect for the radiation treatment. "

"But not perfect enough," she insisted. She continued by saying I should eat – very little fiber, no bran flakes, no oatmeal, no raw vegetables, no whole grain bread or crackers, no prunes or prune juice, no fruit with skin or seeds, etc. No eating pretty much any of my then actual diet!

"So then, what do I eat," I asked.

She responded – white bread, white rice, white pasta, mashed white potatoes, super cooked vegetables with the skins removed, no beans or peas (as they cause gas and would inflate the colon pushing it near the prostate area), clear juice, canned fruit and veggies, etc.

I looked at her like she was crazy, and she said, "I'm not your cardiologist and this is just for 8 weeks of radiation."

I told her that I had tried her suggested diet for a recent colonoscopy, and it blocked me up. But she responded that over time it wouldn't do that and would make me regular. She said I just needed to trust her.

I kept staring at her thinking, "How could eating a concoction that would produce Elmer's glue in my gut make me regular?"

So, she said, "We want as little waste in the colon as possible, and while fiber helps regularity, the body does not digest fiber so eating lots of fiber makes your stools larger. And we want smaller stools because we want the colon as far away from the radiated area as possible and not nudging against it with a large stool inside."

OK, so now I got that point – small stools.

And then she said, "Oh, there is one more thing. While we want an empty colon, we also want a full bladder. And this is what you need to do: empty your bladder 60 minutes before your radiation appointment and then drink 24-32 ounces of fluid so when you get here, you'll have a full bladder."

OK, but I'm thinking, you have to be kidding me, this is getting unreasonably complicated. My bladder sphincter is already a bit weak from the surgery that removed the prostate last June, and will be further weakened by this radiation therapy, and now I have to drink 3-4 glasses of water just before the therapy which will give me an almost bursting bladder – hey you try it – drink four glasses of water and try to walk around without bending over and crossing your legs or leaking!

And I'm going to ride the express bus down to the therapy. So my brain says, "What is going to happen as I try and down 32 ounces of fluid while bumping up and down and swaying back and forth on a public bus zooming down Lake Shore Drive, and then jerking to four stops on Michigan Avenue, before delivering me to the block I walk down to get to the Northwest Hospital, which is right in the middle of the Michigan Avenue's Magnificent Mile shopping area? Can I make it without leaking??? I better wear dark pants and not khakis! No one told me that radiation therapy would be such a challenge."

In sum: I realized all this was working out a lot differently than I had thought. I was going to have more than my share of interesting, er, challenging, experiences!

I did experiment with the low residue diet before I started radiation. The diet nurse provided me with some papers that showed the fiber content of various foods: fruits, vegetables, cereals, breads and crackers. Protein has no fiber, interestingly. I found canned soups with zero fiber. I found crackers, even tasty crackers, with zero fiber or less than 1 fiber in a 4-cracker serving. English muffins, made with processed white flour, have very little fiber and are tasty. Most fruits have a lot of fiber, but honeydew melon does not so I bought one. I bought Rice Crispies instead of Bran Buds and Rice Chex instead of Shredded Wheat. Both the rice cereals floated on top of the milk in the cereal bowl, showing how much nutrition they provided, but rice has zero fiber, so I was eating the right thing. I decided to have lots of fish as that is easy to digest (and I needed a successful bowel movement every day before 9:30 as my radiation appointment was for 10:30), as is white pasta. Eggs are low in fiber.

Weird though it was, the diet actually worked. I did stay regular, the solid waste was much less, the stools were smaller though more difficult to exit the body. The nurse was right. (Sorry about these gory details but it is part of the story and these details matter, I think.)

Hot flash.

As an update, I sent most of the above several pages to a select few of my friends, as not everyone has a sense of humor even when it's at someone else's (mine in this case) expense. I told them the actual radiation would not start until April 17 and that if anyone asked how I was doing, to tell them I was in good hands. ☺

Here is a helpful reply one friend sent:

> *Yes, one needs to not only laugh but also give up all vestiges of bodily modesty/privacy. Of course, after the novelty wears off, you realize that the nurses have seen it all, countless times, and have no prurient interest in your lower half; they are not titillated and do not discuss your privates while in the other room during the actual zapping. I found them – yes pretty, but more interested in my mind and voice. Stimulating conversation and good stories help break up their tedious routine. After a few weeks, I hit upon the idea of singing a different song to them each day; they loved it, because no patient had ever sung to them before. By the way, I was excited, during my SIM, to realize that I was getting my first tattoo! This*

turned out to be a disappointment, however, because I never could find those permanent dots.

Three more notes about your upcoming daily zaps. First, arriving for my daily appointments with empty colon and full bladder turned out to be less daunting than I expected. The key for me was to do most of my (water) drinking once I'd arrived at the waiting room. Turned out, in my case at least, that a half-full bladder was plenty good enough.

Second, while the nurses move you into the exact position on the table, you will be tempted to help them, by shifting your weight, etc. They will keep telling you not to help them. I'm a professional helper, so I found this instruction hard. Just lay back and let them manipulate you.

Third, as the machine rotates and clanks and hums around you, there's a TV up above, to distract you. Day after day it was this channel that was playing country western songs while the still screen shares information, such as, "DID YOU KNOW that [this musician whom you've never heard of] was born in such-and-such year and has two older siblings?"]. Eventually I found out that I could request a Light Classics version of this same format. And late in my seven-and-a-half weeks of radiation, I discovered I could watch a video of a beautiful bubbling brook. Why, I asked, had I not been told about this latter option? Oh, apologized a nurse, because our women patients are afraid the sound of running water might activate their full bladders...

Actually, I sailed through my 38 radiation treatments — and during the nights got used to throwing off blankets and changing out of soaking wet night shirts — and had only minor experiences of diarrhea, no urethral burning sensation, and no skin burning. I also was able to exercise a lot while also ignoring dietary recommendations. My community of Hope Lodge (at the Mayo Clinic in Rochester, Minnesota) friends began to joke that I wasn't really sick but a spy for the American Cancer Society.

What did come as a surprise to me, over the weeks and months after coming home, was the gradual realization that the side effects of these therapies are real and very slow to overcome, namely, reversing the weight gain and regaining stamina. Lupron is strong stuff: a year and a half after my six-month shot, I am still experiencing hot flashes at night, though much milder, fewer, and less distinct. I've sent in two blood samples, at four-month intervals, and was happy to learn that my PSA has remained negligible and that testosterone is beginning a slow comeback.

E.B., Minnesota

Eleanor arrived back in Chicago on Saturday, April 13. We were scheduled to have lunch with my Naperville-based brother and his wife on Sunday. But it snowed 8 inches that day! Welcome to spring in Chicago! ☹ So, we canceled and drove out the next Sunday when it was sunny and warm.

At the beginning of the week I began in earnest preparing for the onset of radiation therapy on Wednesday.

First Radiation Treatments

My initial appointment was for 2 pm but I was told to arrive 15 minutes early as it was my first time and it might take a few minutes to explain to me the process for the next what I thought would be 40 visits. I had been eating the "low residue" diet for about ten days and could vouch for the fact that it was "low residue"; my stools were not only smaller but also fewer. I guess when you eat things that your body digests, and recall fiber is not digested, elimination is mainly liquid. At least I figured my colon would be in shape for the radiation.

I also followed their directions in terms of filling my bladder. I was about to burst at the seams when I arrived. At one pm, one hour before the appointment this first day, I completely eliminated as much as I could. Then I started drinking water; I drank two glasses at home, hopped on the bus (I was wearing dark pants but didn't bring a towel) and drank two more glasses on the way to the hospital. That's 32 ounces; try doing that in a half hour sometime and hop around without wetting your pants. The bus did bump up and down and sway back and forth as it barreled down Lake Shore Drive, and it did make four jerky stops before dislodging me one block from the hospital. I could feel that my bladder was full – believe me. I slowly walked to the hospital, bypassing a lovely fountain that was gurgling a spray of water, and when inside the hospital proceeded directly to the Radiation Oncology suite – hoping I'd get radiated quickly and would make it through before my bladder exploded after the full treatment.

I was greeted by another young nurse who led me back to a changing room; I was told to remove my pants and underwear and to put on the gown, tying it in the back. I did as I was told; the gown came to about 7 inches above my knee.

I exited the changing room and the nurse guided me to the Treatment Room C, which was the room where I would receive all my treatments. I approached the table on which I was to lie and was asked if I'd like a warm blanket and once again said, "Yes, thank you." As I lay on the table and the gown creeped up, the blanket was carefully laid over my mid-section. The technicians then pushed up my gown and pushed down the blanket to reveal the three black tats that would guide my placement on the table, to ensure that the radiation zaps hit the right spots.

I was asked to move down, so my feet touched the end of the mold on which I rested the bottom of my legs. The nurses then had to move me back and forth a bit to get me into the correct alignment for the radiation machine. At first and unconsciously, I tried to help them, but as my friend had warned, the nurses told me to stay still and let them do the moving. Finally, I was in the right position. They took an X-ray, which showed both whether my body was positioned correctly and whether my colon was sufficiently empty and the bladder sufficiently full. Dr. John, my radiation oncologist, then reviewed the X-ray and gave the go ahead. And I got the four zaps: one from directly above, one from each side and one from directly below. And that was it; that part took less than five minutes. Piece of cake, it seemed.

After the treatment was completed, the doctor came in to talk, asking if I had any questions. I said we needed to hurry because my bladder was about to burst. He smiled and said, "Next time drink just two glasses of water; that should be sufficient."

I wanted to hug him! I also learned that the treatments would continue every day for six weeks, then there would be a week break, and then two more weeks. He said if my body was tolerating the radiation well, the break could be shorter, as he knew I wanted as much time between the end of the treatments and the beginning of our trip to Europe. At the end of our conversation, he advised me to get some over-the-counter Imodium, which stops diarrhea. "Keep two pills in your pocket during the duration of your radiation treatments, just in case the treatments cause you to have diarrhea, a common side effect."

I also turned to him and said, "Dr. John. I'm curious. Do you ever do just the hormone therapy for someone like me, with the recurrence detected early and the PSA at a low level?"

And he immediately said, "No. Only radiation and surgery are curative. Hormone therapy helps but I always provide the combination treatment, which is highly effective."

Ok, so there was no way I was going to dodge getting 40 zaps of radiation.

He then asked if I had had any problems.

I said, "Well, I couldn't find a urologist in Sarasota to give me the Lupron shot."

He showed surprise and responded, "I have many patients all over the country and they have no problem getting the shot outside of Northwestern Memorial Hospital group."

I said, "Well, I did; I worked through your nurses and they just couldn't get a urologist to do it."

And Dr. John said, "Oh no, you need to use the urologist's nurse."

Thus, I decided that when I needed my next booster, I would go through that nurse to schedule the shot in Sarasota; if it worked that would save me a plane trip back to Chicago, though I always loved being in the Windy City.

I also learned that once every week I would be checked by the nurses and doctor for my vital signs, to make sure my body was not suffering in some way from the radiation.

Hot flash.

On my way back home, I thought about my getting on the table and the blanket. If I had said, "No, I don't need the blanket," it would seem I'd be lying there totally exposed, which, other than perhaps embarrassing, was simply a bit gross, unseemly as it were. Particularly for this first visit, the nurses came back after the initial X-rays and talked to me for a few minutes, explaining how the radiation machine would move around me to provide the zaps, and then the doctor came in after the treatments were completed and also talked with me. My laying there virtually naked and talking as if nothing was unusual seemed a tad untoward, if I did not have the blanket on me.

On my second treatment, though, I learned that this would not happen. The general procedure was the same. I arrived in the Radiation Oncology suite and checked myself in with a card that had a bar code with my name and treatment specifics. My name appeared on a screen in the reception area, showing that "Allan O" had "Checked-in." When it was time for me to get treated, the line with my name turned green and read "Ready." I then walked to the changing room and, after putting on the gown, sat on a chair just around the corner and waited for the nurse to take me to Treatment Room C.

At that second visit, I again was asked if I'd like a warm blanket, and I said, "Yes, thank you." But I noticed that when I sat on the table, as the first step in lying down on it, one nurse carefully put a towel over my mid-section as I turned and lay down on the table, while another nurse almost simultaneously covered me with the warm blanket – which is very comforting as the room (as are most hospital treatment rooms) was chilly. So, I learned that, in fact, one's lower body was always covered, even if one didn't want the warm blanket. But I did want that warm blanket as the treatment room was cool.

This visit went very quickly. The four zaps were provided, and I was up and out in less than 15 minutes. As they say, I was in and out in a flash ☺. Other than having this procedure once every weekday for the next 38 such weekdays, plus the week break, actually getting the radiation zaps seemed like it would be easy.

I learned, however, that the treatments are not that pro forma for everyone. At my second treatment session, I talked with another man who was getting his fifth treatment. We were sitting on those chairs, short gown to short gown as it were. He was having difficulty getting and holding a full bladder. This day he had an 8 A.M.

appointment, as I did that day. (Though I had requested a treatment time of 11 A.M., my treatment times varied for the first two weeks until my preferred time opened up, which turned out to be 10:30 A.M.) He had started drinking water at 5:45, had consumed 52 ounces by 7:55, and his bladder somehow was not positioned correctly. He was told to wait but finally had to relieve himself, so was facing at least another hour of drinking and getting his bladder into the proper position. His first visits thus were much longer, and he had to go through the process of filling and emptying his bladder more than once.

I am not sure what the issue was, but my point is that everyone is different and that while at that point my treatments seemed to be going well, as they had for other friends, that might not be the case for everyone. I was grateful that my treatments were going smoothly and that I only had to drink 2-3 glasses of water before each appointment; holding "it" after consuming that amount of liquid was not easy but at least was doable for me.

My Ongoing 10:30 Treatments

I had been asked at what time I would like my daily treatments and told that it might take a week or so for my preferred time to open up. That was the case and for the 9th treatment I was able to get my preferred time of 10:30 A.M. This timing would allow me to retain my morning ritual: drink 2-3 cups of coffee, read two newspapers, take my daily morning four-mile walk, shower before bussing to the hospital, get the zaps, and play duplicate bridge at 12:15 two days a week at the downtown Chicago Duplicate Bridge Club, continue with ballroom dance lessons on Tuesday and Thursday early afternoons, and have my afternoons free for the rest of the day. It also would allow me to play my regular 9-hole golf game every Tuesday morning at the Chicago Public Course that bordered Lake Michigan at 40th street North. So other than a daily morning commitment – to save my life as it were – the treatments caused little disruption to me and because up to this time the side effects were modest if any, the treatments seemed easy to handle.

More to the point: chemotherapy – the treatment for many if not most cancers – is very hard on the patient. I was not going to endure anything compared to those who needed chemo. Sure, I was dealing with cancer, but I was not struggling or battling like so many others. Again, as a nurse friend told me, "No man wants to get cancer, but if you do, prostate cancer is the one to get."

Getting the fluid drinking right. It took me several days initially to completely figure out the water drinking routine. Every day I would go through my usual water drinking routine, emptying my bladder around 9:30 and then downing about three plus glasses of water before my 10:30 appointment. Thus, I did have a pretty full bladder when I checked in.

Hot flash.

By the middle of the second week, I was walking about ten blocks to the Bridge Club after my radiation treatment. But the first two times I took that trek I almost didn't make it even though I had thoroughly relieved myself right after the treatment. And when I hit the bathroom at the bridge center, my stream spewed out like a firehose. I thought maybe my bladder sphincter was being weakened by the radiation.

So, at my third weekly "check-up" session with the nurses and doctors, I told them about this problem – first the oncology nurse, second a new female resident, both of whom looked at me quizzically, and then Dr. John, who immediately said, "Don't drink so much water." And that worked and I recalled my above friend who found out that drinking the water after he arrived in the waiting area actually had worked for him.

It also dawned on me that I was downing much more fluid than I realized. I usually arose about 6 A.M. I made coffee and sat down for about two hours to read several newspapers. I'd start with one cup of hot water, followed by 2-3 cups of coffee (half regular and half decaf) and sometimes another cup of hot water. Then I'd have my daily bowel movement, during which I'd eliminate some of the fluid. After I'd go on the 4-mile walk. After that, I'd shower, eat a small breakfast with about a cup of milk with my cereal, urinate as much as I could at 9:30, hop on the bus and drink another 16 ounces of water. By this time, I would have downed 48-56 ounces of fluid in a 3 ½ hour time span, but not eliminated it all.

So, I began reducing the water I drank on the bus and that helped. I did have to "go" right after the treatment, but I could walk to the bridge center without having to look for an empty alley to relieve myself. I did arrive for treatment with a full bladder that needed relief quite soon after the treatment. No problem if everything was on time.

Hot flash.

Treatment Room C delayed 30 minutes. But everything wasn't always on time. One day I walked into the Radiation Oncology Suite all "watered up," as it were, and the screen displayed a note that "Treatment Room C is 30 minutes delayed." Oh, no. I sat there for about fifteen minutes and couldn't hold it and went to the nearest bathroom and relieved myself. I was able to stop before it all drained out, and I quickly drank another 8 ounces, but at that point I realized I might need a contingency plan.

Indeed, for the next two weeks my treatment room was delayed 20-30 minutes every day. Some of the time it was for men in the last 2-3 weeks of treatment when, I was soon to learn, the full bladder issue was much more critical. By the time my line turned green with the "Ready" sign and I approached the (un)dressing room, I often found two to three men drinking water and walking around to speed the water's descent into their bladder. Since these men were at the last stages of their treatments, and had gone through the undressing and putting on the gown routine many times, they also had eliminated the not-so-easy step of fastening the back of their gown, so as they paced up and down the hallway they'd flash their skinny asses as they walked by, as if anyone was interested! TMI?

By this time, I had learned that I needed to hedge my bets on the water. Since I had now realized that I could be downing 48-56 ounces of liquid before arriving at the hospital, I began to cut down on the water I drank on the bus, and sometimes – as my friend had done – began drinking the last cup or so of water after I checked in – and knew if my treatment would be on time or delayed. If the delay was over 15 minutes I waited until about 10:15 before drinking additional water, as once at about that time when I was fully "liquidized" the screen flashed a 30-minute delay.

I also discovered about this time that the empty bowel and full bladder requirement was not so critical for my first six weeks of radiation treatment. All this diet and water drinking work for nothing??? Almost drowning from drinking so much water and to no avail?? What I learned was that the treatment area for the first 5-6 weeks of radiation was broader than just my prostate area. Though the doctors believed that the cancer cells that had escaped my prostate sac were probably in the area where the prostate had been, they also knew that those cells could have moved outside of that small area so directed the radiation beam onto a broader area of my groin to get those possible more errant cells. And, yes, men who did not do a great job of emptying their bowel and filling their bladder often had more side effects at this point – burning sensation when urinating and diarrhea – so exerting effort to get them both right was rewarded. But not as critical as for the last weeks of treatment.

I was told that during the last weeks of radiation, all the power of the beam would be focused on just my prostate area and every day – before the treatment – the technicians would take an X-ray to make sure the colon and bladder were properly positioned and if not, would ask me to drink more liquid to make that happen. The bottom line: getting the bowel and bladder for the first weeks of treatment was good practice for the need to get them absolutely right for the last weeks of treatment. As a doctor friend of mine said, "The radiation technicians want a predicable anatomy when they buzz your groin."

Toward the end of the fourth week, I also began to have bleeding from hemorrhoids during a bowel movement. I had had modest bleeding every several months for many years before the onset of cancer, but the issue would last a day or two and then subside. And I had never been "public" about this issue. Try casually mentioning in some conversation that you bleed every now and then when you have a bowel movement. Do this only if you want the conversation to stop!

But after seeing blood for a week, which had never lasted this long, I somewhat reluctantly decided I needed to "go public" and tell the doctor and nurses during the regular weekly check-up session after the radiation treatments.

Once again, I was forced to discuss a pretty private issue with, not strangers as I was beginning to know all those who provided me the treatment services, but still not my best friends. I actually thought the radiation treatments could be harming my rectum and causing or worsening the bleeding symptoms. So, when the first nurse asked if anything had changed, I said,

"Yes, during bowel movements I have been bleeding from hemorrhoids for the past week."

She immediately responded, "Get Preparation H; it should deal with this issue quickly," and asked me if I knew what a hemorrhoid was. She continued, "It is a swollen blood vessel that periodically bleeds when a person has a bowel movement and Preparation H reduces the swelling." Ok, the cure sounded simple enough!

When the new oncology resident arrived, she asked if there was anything new. I also told her about the bleeding. She replied, "Everyone or nearly all people your age have hemorrhoids; they are almost universal." And she said, "If Preparation H doesn't work, we can prescribe a suppository, which will certainly do the trick."

While it took a week, the Preparation H did work. And one more surprising glitch of this journey seemed to be resolved, or at least under control.

Halfway through. At the halfway point, i.e., after 20 treatments, I sent emails to my family and several friends that I was halfway through my radiation treatments, and that so far, I had experienced no major side effects, such as diarrhea. I didn't go into detail on the fluid drinking or some of the other aspects that I had experienced – as in the big picture they were no big deals – and said all seemed to be going well.

Hot flashes – kept coming 3-4 times a day.

The Break

About this time, I learned that I would have a week-long "break" in my eight-week radiation treatment regime. Initially, I was told the break would occur after the sixth week of treatment, i.e., after 30 zaps, but at this time I was told it would occur after five weeks. So, from May 22 to May 29 I would not receive any radiation treatments. This was good news. My wife and I were planning on going to a nice restaurant in our neighborhood to celebrate our 53rd wedding anniversary on May 28 and not having to go through my usual morning process to be ready for treatment meant that I could sleep-in the next day.

A break after five weeks would mean, though, that the bladder and bowel alignment requirements would be more of an issue for three rather than two weeks, so I

93

began to prepare myself for a more explicit regimen to make all this happen as required.

I must add at this point that during the entire radiation treatment process our 90-year-old-historic building and specifically our apartment was having all hot- and cold-water pipes, vents and drains replaced. Since the walls of the building were comprised of plaster on brick and not plaster on two-by-four walls and since all pipes were embedded in the concrete floors, and many pipes were also embedded in the walls in concrete, these renovations were complicated, noisy, dusty, disruptive, dirty and took six weeks for each bathroom and kitchen. Shortly after Eleanor had returned to Chicago, our master bathroom was completed, but we were living through the renovations to our second bathroom.

Then on May 18, we were informed that work on our kitchen would begin on May 21, a week earlier than planned. So just as I was about to enter a treatment stage when the bladder and bowel issues were critical, and thus my diet was even more important, we could not cook at home. We would have to eat most of our meals out, get frozen meals and cook then in the microwave oven, or somehow eat meals that were complimentary to my needs. Not a huge deal nor a high hurdle to surmount but another element with which to deal during the last three weeks of treatment.

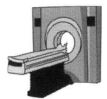

7

The Last Intensive Treatments

During my eight-day break from the first round of radiation treatments, I thought every day about the bowel and bladder issues that would be critical during my last three weeks of treatment. Yes, I was a bit concerned and wanted to have my anatomical parts in the right positions and breeze through the treatments. I did not want to cause delays.

In the next few pages, I provide considerable detail on this issue because even though I thought I had figured out how to handle the bowel and bladder issues, every day seemed to be a challenge. And every day the guys who were having their last three weeks of more intensive radiation treatment talked to each other about how we were dealing with the bladder and bowel issues; some started drinking water at 5 A.M., some took GasX, some took a laxative, some arrived early and then began drinking water, others had different strategies. We all were working on the same issues because if the bladder and bowel were not in the right position/condition we would have to make them so or forego treatment for that day.

Hot flash.

Treatment Room C is delayed 45 minutes. On the first day of the last three weeks of my treatment I awoke at 6 A.M., went through my morning routine of drinking water and coffee and reading the paper, went on a four-mile walk, showered, ate my cereal and at 9:30 boarded that bumping and swaying express bus that delivered me downtown. I actually had drunk five glasses of liquid that morning (two water and three coffee), and while I had relieved myself of some of that liquid, some remained. I drank just a bit of water on the bus ride downtown. At 10 A.M I arrived in the radiation oncology suite for my ten-thirty appointment. The top of the screen read, "Treatment Room C delayed 30 minutes." Good thing I had not consumed a lot of water on the bus.

I checked myself in, slithered into a chair and opened my iPad to work on a crossword puzzle, an activity that had made time go by quickly. I began drinking some more water, even though I could feel I was moving toward the verge of "having to go." I worked on the puzzle for what I thought was a long time, looked up at the clock and only about five minutes had passed. How was I supposed to relax when I knew the bladder issue was key but didn't really know when I'd get into the treatment room? I then noted that there were three people ahead of me for Treatment Room C. Not a good sign. I kept sipping water – I wanted to be ready but not too ready. And continued with the puzzle.

I had drunk about a glass and a half, when the screen suddenly changed to "Treatment Room C delayed 45 minutes!" Oh boy, this initial treatment of the intensive phase of radiation was going to be a real test. In a normal situation, I would have gotten up and relieved myself but that really was not an option. Since I was close to the brink, the time dragged on as I continued to work on the puzzle. But I was beginning to get concerned; I did not want to be one of the guys walking around the hall drinking water and flashing my skinny ass. I wanted my treatment to be provided after the first X-ray. I decided I couldn't concentrate and put the puzzle away – and crossed my legs.

At 11:10 am, my line on the check-in screen finally turned green indicating Treatment Room C was "ready" for Allan O. At that point, I did not hop up and speed down the hall; I couldn't make it that way and stay dry. What I did was I slowly got up and slowly walked to the (un)dressing room, and slowly took off my clothes and slowly put on a gown. I was getting to the breaking point. Any sudden movement would break the dam, so I was moving slowly and carefully.

I sat on the chair for about five minutes, nervously tapping my toes on the floor. Finally, one of the radiation technicians came, apologized for the delay, and asked me how I felt. I said I was about ready to burst and hoping I'd make it through the treatment. She rushed me (slowly) into the treatment room, another person asked if I wanted a warm blanket, I said yes, I slowly got on the table, the blanket was placed over my mid-section and we were ready to go.

The team lined up the beams to the three tats on my lower body, and then said they would first take an X-ray before starting the radiation treatment. I said, "No problem." So, I lay there, holding it, and the machine made a 360-degree rotation around my body.

Then one of the technicians said over the speaker, "OK, we have the X-ray and now we must wait for the doctor to review it."

And I'm thinking, "The doctor isn't back there?"

So, I asked, "And where is the doctor?"

The technician shouted back, "He's in the building somewhere. He'll be here shortly."

Really? I was about ready to drown from "holding it" and now progress was halted until the doctor gave approval and he "was in the building somewhere?" OMG. I did a couple of hard Kegels.

Finally, word came that the doctor had arrived and given approval to provide the more intensive radiation treatment. Immediately the machine whirred and did another, slow, 360 rotation around my body, "zinging" me the entire time. When the machine quit turning, I started to move but the technician said, "No, stay still. The machine will do that again." And about 15 seconds later, the machine began whirring again, reversed itself, and gave me another 360-degree groin buzz.

Shortly after, the team came in and said, "OK, we are done."

I got up off the table and rushed to the nearest bathroom. As I was leaving the treatment room one of the technicians said, "By the way, your bladder and bowel were perfect." Thank heavens for that, but my goal now was to make it to the nearest toilet and relieve myself. I did make it. For over a minute clear liquid spewed forth like a fire hose showing that indeed my bladder was pretty full.

So, the first intensive treatment was a success if somewhat of a challenge. I concluded, though, that I needed a contingency plan for every day. I decided that I should arrive around 10 am every day; if the treatment was on schedule, I thought that provided sufficient time to down 1-2 glasses of water and be ready for the radiation treatment. But if there was a delay, then I could wait to consume the appropriate amount of liquid.

I should also add that during the break I had decided to depart a bit from the low residue diet. Eating so little fiber simple wasn't good for regular and easy bowel movements. I began to have my regular Bran Buds with my morning cereal, and during the break that got me back to a predictable and easy schedule. And since the technician said my anatomy was in good shape for the first intensive treatment, I decided to continue that practice – concluding that for me, as long as I had a morning bowel movement before going to treatment, the bladder was the more critical issue, and I thought I had pretty much figured out the bladder issue.

Hot flash.

The best laid plans. After concocting the plan to ensure the bladder was appropriately full and the bowel appropriately empty, I approached the second day after the break with optimism. I went through my full morning routine, including drinking 4 glasses of liquid, taking a 4-mile walk, and having a bowel movement. I boarded the express bus at 9:30 and arrived at radiation oncology suite at about 9:55, close to my ten o'clock goal. Surprise! There not only were no delays, there were no people using Treatment Rooms A and D, and only two using Treatment Room C, and both of those were already flashing "ready." I checked-in (realizing later I should have waited to check-in after I had drunk a sufficient amount of water and given it time to filter down into the bladder), and began downing water, as I had consumed no water on the bus. It takes about 20-30 minutes (actually 45 I learned a couple days later) for liquid to reach the bladder. I was hoping I'd be OK. But at 10:15 my line turned green and read "ready." So, I arose, walked to the (un)dressing room, put on my gown and sat in the chair, thinking I'd be out of there before my initial appointment time.

Almost immediately, a nurse came and said the team was ready. I got on the table, the team lined up the beams with the tats, and proceeded to take the initial X-ray. The nurse came back with a long face, so I knew something wasn't right. There was a two-pronged problem. She said I had gas in my lower intestine, and I needed to get rid of it; she also said my bladder was only 60 percent full and needed to be fuller, so I was problematic on both issues.

She walked me into the hall and said, "I know it is difficult to get rid of gas while not also emptying your bladder."

She continued, "It is hard to relieve the back side without also relieving the front side."

I knew that already, because I had already started to think about how this new process was going to play out – and began to realize I was going to be here for a while. She said some guys pace the halls trying to have the gas drop naturally; I said I had already taken a four mile walk so didn't think that would be too successful. She said other guys get on their knees and push their rears in the air and that sometimes worked.

Actually, the objective here was for me to "fart" on demand. Yes, I had done that as a teenager, even "lighting" the fart as it blew out of my arse. But I didn't have a full bladder then. And I wasn't a teenager anymore. Nevertheless, I needed to get rid of the gas – fart on demand as it were, or I wouldn't get my second intensive treatment.

I walked the halls for about ten minutes; nothing happened. I then went to the restroom, got on my knees, raised my rear, and sort of prayed for a fart – feeling a bit embarrassed for making this prayer wish, but a fart was what I needed. God would forgive me if such a prayer was inappropriate. And miraculously, I felt the need to expel gas. I immediately got on the toilet not knowing what else would be expelled. And I did release gas but couldn't hold the bladder, so both back and front sides got relief.

Right away, I started drinking more water, and walking the halls – trying to keep the back of my gown together so I wasn't flashing my skinny ass – and feeling that now I was causing a delay in Treatment Room C. Ah well, nothing I could do about it – except expel the gas and fill the bladder. Man, I had never concentrated so much on these processes!

And then – again surprisingly – I felt another urge to release gas, hurried back to the restroom, sat on the toilet, and this time held my "thing" to prevent my bladder from totally going empty. And it worked; the gas blew out and that was it. I kept drinking water.

When I returned to the chairs outside the (un)dressing room, there were two other guys sitting there, getting themselves prepared as well. One was working on his bladder, I confessed I had worked on gas in my intestine, and the other guy was simply waiting for radiation for a brain tumor – which put my situation and the situation for the other man there for recurrent prostate cancer into context. We had super high prospects for being cured; dealing successfully with a brain tumor was much more complicated and a cure was more tenuous.

Finally, the technician came, took me in, put me on the table, covered me with the warm blanket, moved everything down to expose the tats, lined up the tats with the beam, and took the initial X-ray. All was OK. So, the machine whirred and did a 360 counterclockwise rotation around my groin area, stopped for about 15 seconds, and then whirred and did a 360 clockwise rotation. And my second treatment was completed.

I asked the nurse how my anatomy looked – and she said, "Perfect, no gas and a full bladder," flashing me the OK sign.

I walked out at 11:30, a good one hour late. ☹ My conclusion at that point: every day could be different. I had no idea why I had so much gas. And I decided that I also would not "check-in" until after I had downed 1 ½ glasses of water after arriving, so at least my bladder would be ready for the zap.

Hot flash.

"Potty conversations." I shared all these trials and tribulations with my lovely wife, including the low residue diet, which still largely determined our dinner. And this sharing of course led to some what might be called "potty" conversations. Since my stools were smaller and often loose, I asked my wife if she was experiencing the same thing. You might be surprised that we had never before discussed the size and quantity of our stools. I also shared my strategies for filling my bladder, and her response was that she didn't think she could down that much liquid and still stay dry. At any rate, my bowel and bladder challenges began to influence what we talked about during my last three weeks of treatments. And it helped as she worried with me as I tried to address these issues every day and morning so my treatments could be successfully provided.

Why Treatment Room C was delayed so often in the morning. After about six days of consistent delays for Treatment Room C, during the early treatment phase, I asked one of the receptionists if mid-morning was a time when there usually were delays. Her response:

"Actually, no. Mornings had been quite free flowing with few delays. The delays usually occurred in the late afternoons."

I was curious. When I got to the treatment room, I asked the technicians about the delays (thinking they were primarily guys not having their bowel and bladder conditions appropriately ready for treatment).

One of them said, "No, it is not the guys. In the early morning we treat children with cancer; they often are sedated so they will remain still. And sometimes there are difficulties or complications and it takes longer to provide their radiation treatments."

Wow ☹ Kids with cancer. That broke my heart and made me feel sad. So, I said, "No problem ever with me in terms of delays. Take all the time you need; those kids need all the attention you can provide."

And as with the man who was being treated for a brain tumor, whatever challenges us guys with prostate cancer had, our chances of being cured were quite high, and with respect to children, we all already had lived a full live, and all those kids needed to be cured and deserved a long life as we all had experienced.

Your bladder is not full. I continued to arrive at the Radiation Oncology suite at about 9:55 to gauge the status of Treatment Room C. As just noted, it was delayed just about every day. And my bladder strategy was working. But then at about my 7th intensive radiation treatment, and after the initial X-ray to determine if my bowel and bladder were in the appropriate condition, the technician came back and said,

"Your bladder is only 50 percent full. You need to drink another glass or two of water and let it drain down into your bladder before we can provide the treatment."

So, I went out in the hall, got my glasses of water, and began drinking. And it worked.

After 20 minutes, the technician said, "Let's try it again."

We did and everything went well.

Every day I went through the same routine – drinking 1-2 cups of water in the morning as well as three cups of coffee, going on my walk, getting to the Radiation Oncology suite at about 9:55, and then downing about 2 cups of water. And most of the time I was fully prepared bladder-wise.

I did the same thing for my 8th intensive treatment. When I arrived, I had a small bowel movement, even though I had had one at home earlier. And I lost some but not a lot of bladder fluid.

I immediately went to the waiting room and found no delay for Treatment Room C and the systems were "ready" for everybody checked-in for Treatment Room C. I did not check in right away. I began drinking water and stayed standing while doing so. I drank a full 2 ½ cups of water, and then checked in. I got another glass and drank it while talking to two other men, one of whom was getting his last treatment this day. At about 10:30 the line on the screen for "Allan O" turned green and read "Ready" and I said good-bye to my friends and sauntered down the hallway to the (un)dressing room. I took my clothes off and put on the gown. But I didn't feel an urge to "go."

The technician came and got me, put me on the table, and took the initial X-ray and came back and said, "Your bladder is pretty much empty. When was the last time you went to the bathroom?"

I said I did a bit at 10 o'clock but had downed 4-5 glasses of water since.

And she said, "Well, you must be dehydrated." Another new thing!

I couldn't imagine why I'd be dehydrated. The previous day, I actually had consumed more fluid than usual, and had drunk more than my usual number of cups of water that morning. Nevertheless, I downed another 3 glasses. I waited for three more people to be treated – one for a tumor at the end of his tongue, one for breast cancer, and another a fellow with recurrent prostate cancer, who also worked each day to get his bowel and bladder in appropriate condition. The bladder issue for this man was even more challenging as he had never regained bladder control after his prostate surgery so when he poured water down his throat some leakage occurred that simply was beyond his control.

For me, even after downing 8 glasses of water that morning, I didn't feel a strong urge to "go." But about 50 minutes after my 10:30 appointment, the technicians accompanied me back to the treatment room, took the X-ray, found that my bladder had finally filled, and provided the intensive radiation treatments.

I rushed to the bathroom after the treatments were completed and had one of those "fire hose" elimination experiences. And I expected that I would not make the 10-block walk to the Bridge Club where I was going for an afternoon of bridge playing. So, I walked five blocks to a MacDonald's, ordered a burger, and found the bathroom while I waited for my order to be filled. Another fire hose stream. And then I walked another four blocks to a diner just a half block from the Bridge Center. I rushed in, the receptionist asked,

"Can I help you?" and I said,

"I need to use the bathroom," as I rushed by.

And another fire hose stream. And I even stopped in the bathroom after I got to the Bridge Club. So, the 8 cups of water were indeed going through my system. And I had just experienced another unpredictable treatment scenario.

As I had previously concluded, every day, it seems, could be different. Though this created some uncertainty each treatment day, I was grateful for the care that was being taken before the radiation treatments were provided. In the earlier days of radiation, all these precautions were not always taken and sometimes the radiation beams caused harm to the colon/rectum. Those unintended effects had now been virtually eliminated and it was due to a combination of more targeted radiation beams themselves, lining up the radiation machine to the three tats to ensure accuracy in where the beams hit, and insuring that the bladder was full and the bowel empty before any radiation treatment was provided (both helping to ensure that the rectum was sufficiently far enough from the radiated prostate area so the beam would not cause harm to the colon).

Hot flash.

By this time, I was beginning to see the end – I had only 8 more treatments before my radiation regimen would be completed. While I felt I was in good care and the team – my doctor, the radiation technicians and the nurses in the radiation oncology suite – were terrific, I was wanting this to be over.

Continuing bladder issues. When my bladder was not sufficiently full for my 8th treatment, one of the radiation technicians said,

"You need to consume the water 45 minutes before your scheduled treatment time; it takes that much time to filter through your body and into the bladder."

So, I started to arrive earlier, and began to drink water much earlier. Moreover, during the last week there were no delays in Treatment Room C so my scheduled treatment time of 10:30 became quite predictable and I needed to be ready by then.

Without going into more detail, I was successful about every other day. It all worked when I was able to consume 20 ounces of water by 9:45 but other things intervened so I was not able to implement even this simple strategy. For example, everything was on time one day and then when I got to the hospital, I had a case of the runs at 10 am and didn't have sufficient time to refill the bladder.

Nevertheless, the radiation technicians were always helpful, cheerful and supportive. They never chided me for not being ready, probably knowing that all of us were doing what we could to make sure our anatomy was appropriately positioned for the treatments.

The End is in Sight

I also found out during this last week that I was going to get only 39 treatments. My doctor said the standard was 38 treatments, and the number for each individual ranged from 38 to 40. My MRI showed one suspicious area near the seminal vesicle to which he wanted to give an extra zap and that was why I was getting 39 treatments. All this was exciting news; I would now finish on Tuesday of the next week and not Wednesday, and believe me, at this point we all were counting the days.

I also learned at this time that I was to be on hormone treatment (the Lupron shots) for two years. Although there is some uncertainty as to the needed length of the hormone treatment, my doctor said that at the present time two years was the standard. So, I would have Lupron shots every four months until October of 2020. Before telling me this, he asked again if I was having any strong reactions to the hormone treatment – hot flashes, swelling of the calves, weight gain, etc. I said that I hadn't; that my hot flashes were really "warm" flashes and that I had no other major side effects (ignoring the shrinkage of my genitals which I, but not the doc, considered major). If I had onerous side effects, he said he would shorten the hormone regime but since I was tolerating the hormones, he felt we should go the full two years.

On the Friday before my last two treatments, I encountered another man finishing his treatments. He stopped and said hi, and I asked him how many treatments he had left.

"Four," he said.

"Congratulations," I replied, "You are almost done."

He replied, "Thanks," and then asked, "How many more do you need?"

I replied, "Two!"

And he said, "Congratulations." Then added, "I hope we never see each other under these circumstances again"

And we both laughed.

We were nearing the end of our treatments, and while in the big picture, we were lucky that these treatments were highly successful and that our cancer likely would be in remission for several years, we also were anxious to end the treatments, move on and hopefully need no more treatments for cancer.

One more point. During my last weekly check-up with my doctor, I asked if I was "cancer free" now that my PSA read zero. (I had learned the latter after I had a check-up with my internist, something that is suggested halfway through radiation treatment to make sure my vital signs were all normal.)

He replied, "No, you are in remission. We won't know for 5-10 years whether you are cured; the likelihood is high that you are cured, but only time will tell."

And these comments squared with what other friends had told me. The combined radiation and hormone treatments are quite effective, but one can say one is "cancer free" only after several years have passed and there is no sign of recurrence.

Warm flash.

The last two treatments. I wanted my last treatments to go without a hitch. So, on Monday I decided to arrive early and drink all my water by 9:45. I hoped on the bus at 9:30 and drank 2 ½ cups of water by 9:45. I felt good; I should be "on the verge" by the time of my appointment. I got to the Check In area and sat for a while, doing my crossword puzzle. It was about 10:10. I was beginning to "feel the urge." Good, but it was a bit too soon. I sat there hoping I'd get the go signal soon. The check-in screen turned green and "Ready for Allan O."

I got up, slowly walked to the (un)dressing room, put on my gown, and sat in the chair, still feeling a strong "urge to go." I clearly had sufficient water in my bladder. The technician came and said the team was ready, I entered the treatment room, hoped on my table, the team checked that the radiation beams were lined up with my tats, and then took the initial X-ray. All was good. The machine whirred once around counterclockwise, stopped for about fifteen seconds, and then shirred around once clockwise. The next to last day was successful.

But I had to run to the restroom to relive myself with a fire hose stream, and every 20 minutes for the next hour I also let out a fire hose stream. Though my timing was off a bit, I certainly had consumed sufficient amounts of water and the bladder was more than full for the treatments.

On the last day, I actually played 9 holes of golf on the Chicago public course by the lake, ten minutes from my home and halfway to the hospital. Our round ended at 9:30, I hoped on the car and drank two cups of water by 9:55. I parked and got myself to the Radiation Oncology suite. No delays! Good. I waited until 10:20 to check-in and almost immediately the screen turned green and "Ready for Allan O." I was feeling the urge to go.

As I walked by the two receptionists on my way to the (un)dressing room, both said, "Last day, right? Congratulations!"

Another person who was being treated for a brain tumor asked if he could join me at The Gong after my treatment, and I said, "I'd be honored."

I took off my clothes and put on the gown, and sauntered to the waiting area, now really feeling the "urge." Good, that meant my bladder was full and the treatment would be provided on the first try. The technicians came to accompany me to the treatment room, all saying, "Congratulations, this is your last day." I asked if I could get pictures of them with me, and I got two, one with two of the technicians and one with a technician standing by the radiation machine. I got on the table, they lined up the beams with the tats, took the X-ray, said all was OK, and gave me my last treatment.

I was done with my radiation treatments. Hallelujah!

Treatments completed. I wrote a message of thanks and gave it to these technicians who had been so careful, professional and supportive throughout the entire process. I wanted to make sure both the technicians and the nurses knew I was grateful for what they all had done, and I also wanted to poke some fun at some of the things that had happened. Here is what I wrote:

I want to give all of you a huge THANK YOU for everything you have done over the last 9 weeks to guide me through my radiation therapy. I had no clear idea what the treatment would entail, and I approached my first sessions with some wariness. From the very beginning, you all have been exceedingly professional and super helpful – first talking me through the "low residue" diet and how important it was for successful daily treatments (though I will shift back to a higher fiber diet beginning at noon today), second assuring me when my blood pressure was higher than normal after my radiation treatments (which is now moderated by a small dosage blood pressure medication), and then during my last three weeks of more intensive radiation walking me through what I needed to do to eliminate gas from my bowel (I never knew just walking had such wide spread effects) and fill my bladder to capacity (giving it 45 minutes to fill). Even though I was not successful every day in getting everything right on the first try, as it were, I never felt any disappointment from you – only encouragement to keep trying, and with your guidance I was always successful on the second try.

You have a critical job treating people with various types of cancer. For me, you all always were super supportive, friendly, interested in me as a person, careful in providing my treatments, respecting my privacy, insuring that the beams all lined up with my tats (though it would have been cool if I could have had a small rose or a heart or an arrow or something more exotic than a period, but I understand) and professional in everything you did. You made me feel comfortable and guided me through all the processes that resulted in successful treatments.

*I will miss seeing all of you on a daily basis;
thank you for being nurses and radiation
technicians. Your work is very important, and you
do it with aplomb and skill.*

My best to all of you,

I meant every word. This team together with the doctors were saving my life and I wanted them to know I was deeply grateful.

I then walked to The Gong, which each person who completed their treatments was encouraged to strike. The three technicians and the nurses gathered there with me and took some more pictures. It was a nice ending to my 9 weeks of treatment. I was going to miss seeing them and told them so; I also told them I'd always remember them.

I struck the Gong. And that was it. I left to go home.

But when I took the elevator to the second floor, to take the walkway to where I had parked my car that day, I looked in the mirror and wanted to cry. It is hard to put into words my feeling of relief and thanks, and knowing my PSA was zero further cemented my gratefulness. Most patients do not get a PSA reading until two months after treatment; I accidentally got one earlier and knew things could not be better at this point.

Not only were my treatments over but also, I was a very fortunate man to have had very few side effects, and no major side effects. My doctor told me that one patient could not control his bowel movements for two months and was hospitalized during that entire time; and that it took four months to complete the treatments. I had no diarrhea, no constipation, no weight gain, no burning sensation, pretty much nothing. My "hot flashes" were actually "warm flashes," while most men with whom I talked said theirs were strong and caused sweating. Yes, on a few days, my bladder was not sufficiently full, and I had to drink more water and wait for it to fill. I did get fatigued more than usual, but that meant that on some days rather than just an hour nap, I'd take my usual hour nap as well as a half-hour nap. In the big picture, my treatments had been quite straight forward. I got 39 of them, and also continued my other activities – bridge two days a week, dance lessons two days a week, and golf on Tuesday morning. And now my chances of success were well over 95% and my PSA was already reading zero; it could hardly be better.

On Wednesday morning I woke up knowing there would be no treatment. For the past three months – April, May and most of June – the weather in Chicago had been grim – cloudy most days, rain about every other day (May 2019 went down as the wettest day in recorded history), and temperature in the 50s even in mid-June. I wore my down parka for half the days in June! But on this first day after completing the treatments, I awoke to sunshine! I interpreted this as the dawn of a new time for me. My prostate cancer and its treatments – surgery and radiation – were behind me and I was moving forward. This was the dawn of a new day and I was going to enjoy every minute of the rest of my life.

Afterword

I'd like to make a few additional comments about my prostate cancer journey – so far.

First, I am grateful for having good doctors, nurses and technicians. I believe I received state-of-the-art treatment and the teams were professional and supportive throughout the entire process. My chances for a cancer-free future are high.

Second, as noted earlier, in retrospect I believe I should have seen the urologist about two years before I did, at the point when my PSA rose above 4. There are many reasons for why PSA counts can rise, but a reading above 4 in my lay opinion should lead to more analysis – a test for free antigens, and then if those are below 15 percent or some standard level, on to an MRI. And if like my situation the MRI showed possible lesions, then the targeted biopsy guided by the MRI results. The sooner one treats prostate – or any – cancer, the greater are the chances for a cure.

Third, even though I delayed seeing the urologist, I have learned that I probably did not miss the "curative window." When I told my urology nurse that I now believe I should have started the processes with them earlier, she said,

"Don't forget. Prostate Cancer moves very slowly, and you shouldn't worry that you missed the 'curative window.'"

She continued, "You had the surgery, and then the radiation treatments and your PSA is now 0. All these data point to positive long-term results for you."

I still would advise men to continue to get yearly PSA tests and to see a urologist when the number rises above 4.0. Even though I delayed treatment for two years after my PSA rose above 4, I would not have done so if I knew then what I think I know now, but I feel better now knowing that I probably did not miss the "curative window".

Fourth, a note on what all this cost me. Virtually nothing. Nearly every man over 65 has Medicare, which covered all my treatments. And I had a good Medi-Gap policy that paid for charges not covered by Medicare. I did have some co-pays for pills I needed to take, but I virtually had all these treatments at no cost to me. And the pill costs have not yet reached $100. Further, If I can read through the opaqueness of the Medicare statements, and they are not easy to read, I have had between $200,000 and $300,000 worth of treatments. Even a 10 percent copay for that would have been a large number. Further, it is clear from the Medicare statements that Medicare dramatically reduces its reimbursement rates for doctors and nurses but pretty much pays the full tab for drugs and the radiation zaps themselves. So, hats off to the doctors and nurses that treatment prostate cancer patients because they receive payments much lower than they charge.

Finally, I would encourage anyone who desires more detailed, and up-to-date medical information on prostate cancer -- diagnosis, surgery, radiation, potency, side effects, etc. -- to read Patrick C. Walsh and Janet Ferrar Worthington's *Guide to Surviving Prostate Cancer* (New York: Warner Books, 2018).

About the Author

Allan Odden is a retired, professor emeritus from the University of Wisconsin, Madison. He worked in education all his life, first as a teacher in New York City's East Harlem, and then as an education policy analyst with a focus on funding K-12 public schools at the Education Commission of the States, the University of Southern California and Wisconsin. He also worked as an advisor and consultant to 35 state legislators on their public-school funding policies and can claim to have played a key role in getting billions of new dollars to property poor school districts and for students from low income and non-English speaking backgrounds. He has been married to his lovely wife Eleanor for 53 plus years. He has a son who lives in Chicago and a daughter and grandchildren who live in Montreal, Canada.

Made in the USA
Coppell, TX
12 January 2020

14239047R00067